THE BOYS

THE BOYS

OR, WAITING FOR THE

ELECTRICIAN'S

DAUGHTER

John Terpstra

GASPEREAU PRESS ¶ PRINTERS & PUBLISHERS
KENTVILLE NOVA SCOTIA
2005

Their hearts were light
and we tried to live as normal
a life as possible

This book is dedicated to three brothers:

NEIL
also known as Lamaar,
Mercury Morris and Merkee Perkee.

PAUL
a.k.a Lenny, Willie,
Russell, Seal and Bull

ERIC
a.k.a. Otis, an owl; and
Ike "Behind-the-Mike" White, a pig.

It is also dedicated to their parents,
FRAN (Mumphy, Muzzer)
and COREY (Boss, Van and Neil).

And it is dedicated to their sister,
MARY ANN (Mary),
and to their nieces, Katie and Anna
whom they never had the pleasure of meeting,
or nicknaming.

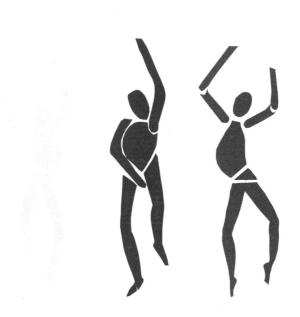

1   There is the story in a nutshell.
     There are the various ways into the story.
     There is the story itself. (There are the stories themselves.)
     There is the question: Whose story is this?

2   The way it usually comes out now, if it comes out at all (as
     it used to; often) is unexpectedly, in the context of other
     conversations.
          The electrician and the nurse meet, they fall in love, and
     marry. Their first child is a daughter. A year later, a son
     arrives. After the first son, two more boys are born; four
     children within six years. By the time the youngest is born,
     the eldest boy is five and has difficulty keeping his balance.
     He frequently falls. His back is curved, distending his belly.
     It's clear something is physically not right.
          They send him to the doctor. The diagnosis, when it is
     made, applies to the second son as well, who has begun
     to show similar symptoms. And his parents can tell, just
     by looking, that the new baby is under the same spell. The
     condition is terminal.
          So begins the long haul through the next twenty years.

3   There are two ways to enter.

One way is through the front door, though it isn't really the front door but the door to the breezeway.

He'd never heard of a breezeway. It is the space between house and garage, a passage approximately one room wide, which may be open or closed at either end. This one was closed on both ends by windows and a door. The windows were jalousies. They worked like venetian blinds: narrow, horizontal glass plates that swivelled open and shut with the turn of a small crank. He'd never heard of jalousies, either.

He'd travelled twelve hours by bus to visit his new girlfriend and her family over the second half of a Christmas break from college. The first half he spent with his own family in Ontario. Staring out the bus window into the darkness of upper New York State he realized that he couldn't remember what she looked like. The abrupt re-entry and immersion into a familial environment which followed their four months together in the intense splendid isolation of college life, hundreds of miles from home, had wiped her face from his mind as effectively as waking dissolves dream.

She was standing beside the family Vista Cruiser as the bus pulled into the small New Jersey town. Ankle-length, grey coat, self-tailored; a product of her Saturday morning apprenticeship to her grandmother. Knitted scarf, grey and red, from her grandmother's own hands. Long, straight hair, hanging down her back. Slender and smiling. A poet. Standing at the gateway to hope.

He enjoyed instant recall.

4 My grandmother sits
and knits.
The carpet snags the wool,
  pulls it
  taut.
The needles slacken, pause,
and pull again,
a timid tug.
She clicks her needles
and stirs the shadows
on the rug.

5 "I couldn't remember what you looked like, either," Mary
Ann said.
 Where did she get this ability to make him feel better and
at the same time not unique?

6 "The boys are lined up, ready and waiting," she said,
guiding the station wagon along the winding roads that
wove between the trees. She turned up yet another hill and
onto a dead-end street at its summit, then onto a dead-end
street that ran off the first, and into the driveway of a long,
white house.
 He climbed the three stairs of the breezeway in naked
fear, saw the door open before him, a father and mother
revealed, and promptly stumbled and fell over the top step,
sprawling at their feet on the carpeted concrete.
 News of the slapstick entrance travelling into the interior
of the house with the speed of a slapshot.

7   Door number two is the previous four months, and the details that emerge as the newly-acquainted pair walk the curb-free streets of the old suburban neighbourhood that surrounds the college they are attending on the outskirts of Chicago.

Family constellations light the sky above them. Stars with a dimly guessed, barely readable effect on their lives.

She has a brother. She laughs. She has two brothers.

He is already confused.

The boys were caught smoking and stealing. They went to the drugstore with Larry and Barry...

Larry and Barry? he asks.

The neighbourhood twins. Larry and Barry were pulling the wagon in case the boys got tired...

Tired?

...and they stole a pack of White Owl cigars, the kind their grandfather smoked, and between the four of them puffed on a few and hid the rest in the gutter above the front door of the house. They were found out when it rained and the cigars began to swell. Boss noticed the brown bulge above the top edge of the gutter.

Boss is their father's nickname, she tells him.

8   She laughed a lot. It was attractive. It was distracting. She told him about the time her brothers were racing down the driveway of the neighbour's house across the street and Paul, the middle one (she has *three* brothers) missed the turn at the bottom, hit a rock and catapulted into the bushes.

"Get me out of here," he said, when the others came running. It was hard to hear him, upside down, hanging in the bushes.

He couldn't get himself out? the new boyfriend asked, wanting to join her laughter. Wanting to laugh for the right reason. Wanting to laugh for the same reason as she.

Of course not, she said.

"Let's go again," Paul said, after they hoisted him out.

9   The boys were lined up, ready and waiting in the bedroom for the arrival of their sister's Canadian boyfriend. Who would, by definition, play hockey. He would be playing hockey with them, at least.

Introductions were brief. A few mumbled, under-the-breath asides about tripping over the threshold, barely audible.

A bit wobbly there.

Johnny's (you don't mind if we call you Johnny, do you?) too light on his feet.

Trying to impress us?

He wasn't sure that he was hearing what he was hearing. Unbeknownst to him, in displaying so extravagantly a physical awkwardness, his fall over the threshold had instantly endeared him to them.

Their chairs were positioned two on one side, one on the other, wheels locked. The passage between them was open at one end, closed at the other by a closet door. A breezeway for scoring. The closet's open doorway acted as goal mouth. Where the Canadian would stand.

Paul and Eric sat side by side. Eric, farthest from the net, passing ahead to Paul, who drop-passed the puck back to his younger brother at the blue line for a slapshot.

The slapshot. Their sticks were authentic, but miniaturized; the puck, the plastic cap of an aerosol can. Surprising, the wallop that such a light object can pack.

He scores.

Got one past the Canuck.

Didn't even break a sweat.

Neil sat opposite the two, wielding instead of a wooden stick a golf club, a 3-iron, which allowed his shots to be based as much on momentum as on muscle. The pendulum effect. The boys set him up for a shot, positioning the puck for his swing. Calculating the trajectories. With much conversation.

He shoots.

The follow-through caught the goaltender off guard. The upswing of the club after it made contact with the lid making contact with his shin.

An accident.

The second time, the glinting eyes and conspiratorial grins were unavoidable, but the hockey player from the north still felt compelled to play humble guest, well-mannered rookie.

The third time, he howled. The response they were looking for. That broke the ice. From that point on, the louder he howled the better the boys liked it. The better they liked it....

They scored. He scored.

10   There are more than two ways in.

    There is falling into conversation one evening twenty-five years after the bedroom hockey game, at a campground in rural Ontario, campfire blazing, songs sung. The initial establishing of who-are-you, where-from, in the ethno-religious, continental web to which both conversants belong causes one of the strands to vibrate. The woman he has just met informs him that she has just returned from New Jersey, where the boys came up in conversation. She'd been talking after church with someone who lived across the street from Mary Ann's family–the neighbour from whose driveway Paul was pitched into the bushes.

    She goes on to say that she entered into her line of work because of the boys, because of Eric specifically. Let's not call it a line of work. Rather, a vocation. She heard the first whispers of her call already in third grade, she said, from being in the same class with Eric, from watching how he was treated by the teacher. The clumsiness, lack of balance, the falling over and needing help to get up: all this extra attention the nine-year-old required was a teacher patience-tester, an irritant. The teacher let the irritation show.

    Seeing her classmate punished for displaying the symptoms of his disease eventually led the campfire stranger into the field of special education.

    He stared into the flames. *They live.*

11   For all this was long ago. The story ended. He does not expect others to remind him. Expects much less that a

stranger will have a part in it, or that it will be a living part of her life. The family of mother, father, daughter and three sons that he visited during a college Christmas break a quarter of a century ago survives only in the person of the woman whose face he could not recall on the bus, in the photographs that hang on their walls.

To outlive. To continue to live *after or in spite of*.

There has been no family reason to return to New Jersey since her mother died and they sold the home, five years ago.

12   There are many ways to enter, and inside is where they live, where she has always lived.

13   We did return, at last, to Mary Ann's home state, to visit a friend who was spending a semester in research at Princeton. We arranged to visit the neighbours who lived across the street from her family, although the couple no longer lived across the street but across the Hudson River from Manhattan, on the Jersey shoreline. From their condominium balcony they could gaze across the water at the toothless gap at the south end of the island, where the twin towers of the World Trade Center had stood only two months earlier.

On the Sunday morning of our weekend trip we returned, too, to Mary Ann's hometown, and attended her childhood church. We drove past the family house, which had been added to and remodelled by its new owners. We stopped at the drugstore of the boy's White Owl caper, now a specialty food shop, which stood at the top of the hill on the town's main street. From that vantage Lower Manhattan is visible. The building of the towers began not long before Mary Ann and I met. We watched them grow during visits home.

Compare and contrast: the building of the twin towers and one family's experience.

We also visited the neighbour's eldest son, Dennis, and his family, who lived at the bottom of the hill. Dennis was a year younger than Eric, the youngest of Mary Ann's three brothers. He'd pushed Eric's special, caretaker-constructed chair-on-wheels through the school hallways, and donated a lot of his time to entertaining the troops, as it were. Acting as surrogate legs and arms. Performing acts of humour and outrage for their entertainment. Getting into trouble by following their prompts.

He chopped a tree down in the front yard, at their urging. And turned to see his father, and Boss, standing behind him. Paul and Eric laughing in the background.

He rode his dirt bike into their house, down the hallway and into Paul and Eric's bedroom, before turning and heading down the hall into Neil's room.

He shot a puck, indoors, a real puck, not the plastic cap of an aerosol can, that went through the bedroom wall, to the hoots and hollers of the riot-inciting threesome. And was chased out the front door for that one, by Mumphy, with a broom.

Mumphy was their mother's nickname.

Now Dennis spent his own days in bed, having over the past five years become apprenticed to fibromyalgia. The disease had taken over his and his family's life. The strain of the disease and of Dennis's unknown future was apparent.

He kept a photo of the boys on his bedroom dresser, he said, to give himself encouragement.

He wanted to know, "All those years in wheelchairs, and in bed. Did they have a lot of pain?"

14   Whose story is this?

15   PLAY-BY-PLAY
An Introduction to the Tedium of Artistry

How Eric shoots baskets.

With a nerf ball: a foam rubber sphere the size of planet Earth, if Jupiter swishes through hoops and Mercury orbits the infield diamond.

In the front hall. Through a basket attached to a masonite backboard attached to the door. From behind a free-throw line at the end of the hallway carpet, five feet out.

Brakes locked. Elbows on the arms of the chair.

The ball is placed in his lap.

He lobsters the sponge-sphere with the thumb and fingers of his right hand, clamps tight, then dips his head downward and shimmies hand and wrist over his crew-cut head until ball and arm are behind his neck, then, using the left arm to help push off, bolts himself upright, throws his upper body weight into heaving backward, and is in position: head cocked, down a little, to the left, right arm bent behind the head, the ball resting on his left shoulder.

He eyes the net, sidelong.

The fluidness that follows is of the pitcher's mound, as

he goes into motion, eyes the net, lifts his head and throws his body against the back of the chair, then hurls himself forward, arm following, loose-jointed as a pitcher. And launches the ball.

Swish.

His spent right arm flops down between his legs, torso following halfway, as though the player is taking a small bow.

Labouriously, incrementally, he works his way up to a sitting position again, elbows again on the chair arms, as the ball is retrieved and placed on his lap.

Replays the routine. Times thirty.

Anything less than a ninety-six percent shooting average annoys him.

16   How Paul does it. With less physical heft working on his behalf. From his living room chair. Using a tennis ball.

Same motions in acquiring the ball, but with an able teammate providing the motor power, placing his arm behind his head, feeding the ball to his hand.

He shoots, from three feet out, into the cannister the balls are sold in: a slim, metal tube that holds three. The tube held by the teammate, at floor level, angled toward the thrower.

He waits. Concentrates.

The lanky, universal-jointed limbs of him. A slumped marionette.

He throws his torso forward, slings his arm over his head and at the precise moment in the arc downward, releases the ball.

Voop.

The ball is sucked into the tube. His average hovers above seventy percent.

Meanwhile, unable to stop his body's momentum, he continues an exaggerated bowing, may have to be caught, held, in order to prevent somersaulting into a heap on the floor. The boy who was hurled into the bushes.

Head hanging between the knees, looking back, he can see the length of the house to the kitchen, notice the gum under the seat. (There is no gum under the seat.)

He can't see what he wants to know.

Did it go in? his only concern.

17 The three, together, in the living room. Fraternal triumvirate.

Merkee, what's your choice? (*Merkee* is Neil's nickname.)

Will it be Stratomatic, Scrabble or Triominos?

Deferring to their elder, the one who goes before them, his wheelchair stationed at the card table.

Or TV?

18 *Dear God, you're kidding. All three?*

This is the usual response. The historical response, of someone first hearing about the brothers.

What is the young couple's response to the news that each of their sons has the terminal disease that the eldest of the three is showing only the first signs of at age five?

We don't know. We (their daughter and son-in-law) never asked.

19 Frances Marie de Puyt, also known as Mumphy, grew up in the same small town where she later lived with her husband and children. The middle child of three. Her parents bought a building lot on Hill Street soon after they married, and hired a carpenter. Many young couples in the 1920s did the same. Fran's aunt and uncle lived next door.

A frame-built home, storey-and-a-half structure, with a street-facing dormer above a screened front porch, and wooden lap siding. Modestly proportioned but on a generous property. A long, narrow driveway ran from the street to a garage with two swing doors in the backyard. No fences separated the neighbours. Chickens were cooped in a pen behind the garage, for their eggs, and later for the pot. A large vegetable garden flourished in the back too, bordered by berry bushes.

The town lay within a certain radius of New York City, and the space between it and the neighbouring towns was slowly beginning to fill in. An organic form of suburbia, that retained a strong rural feel.

Fran's mother, Clara, ran the household and family life in general. Her father, Marinus, commuted daily into New York City, by bus, train and subway, one and a half hours each way, for thirty years.

Her brother and sister both moved out of state after high school graduation, and marriage. Fran found office work in Paterson, a textile city where many Dutch immigrants had settled earlier in the century. Later, she entered nurses' training.

20   In winter, the Hill Street kids tobogganed down the long, gentle slope that gave their street its name.

As a toddler, Frances had slid past her future husband's house. This is part of the family lore. The romance, in a family otherwise short on romance.

21   Cornelis Adriaan Vande Ree, also known as Boss, was born in the Netherlands. His family immigrated to the United States in the early 1920s, when he was two years old, and lived for a time three doors down from the de Puyts. A few years later they returned to visit the old country, and were stranded there by the stock market crash of 1929. The outbreak of World War II further delayed their return to the States.

Corey spent most of the war interned in a German labour camp. He returned home from Berlin on foot after the liberation with one personal possession, a radio. He later regretted having decided to carry it rather than his diary and the book in which were written the names and addresses of the men he spent time with in the camp.

Using his licence as a radio operator, he joined the Dutch merchant marine after the war, travelled to, among other places, Indonesia, then still a colony of the Netherlands, and after a few years decided to return to the United States.

22   Corey began working toward his licence as an electrician. At a roller rink one Saturday evening, he and the toddler on the sled became reacquainted. Fran had recently graduated as a licenced practical nurse. They married, and moved into

the upstairs apartment of a house in Prospect Park, a town next door to Paterson.

Mary Ann was born first, and named after a character in a radio soap opera her mother listened to. An orphan girl. Fran liked the sound of the little girl's voice.

There is a black and white photograph of the electrician and his daughter. He is carrying a high chair, with Mary Ann seated in it. They are at the bottom of the stairs to the apartment. She stares up at the camera. He has eyes only for her.

23 Corey's parents, Walter and Caterina, his two brothers and three of his four sisters had previously returned to the States and were living in the same area of New Jersey. One sister, the eldest child in the family, Co (short for Jacoba), immigrated last.

On Co's first night in the new country, after her six children had been settled into bed in her parents' home, she came downstairs to find her parents putting on their coats, as if to leave.

"Where are you going?" she asked.

"Home," they replied.

"You *are* home," she said.

"No, *you* are. This is your home now." They closed the door behind them and walked across the yard, to the smaller house Walter had recently built for this surprise.

24 Caterina died a few months later.

Within the year, Walter remarried. His new wife was Alice, a widow.

Walter and one of his sons, Lauw, were in business together as masons. Alice was Lauw's mother-in-law, and now his stepmother. Together Lauw and his father had built the house for Co's surprise. Now, they drove the truck around the corner and built a house for Walter and Alice: single-storey, concrete block, with a smooth, white stucco exterior.

25   Walter pointed out the view from his new living room window to Corey and Fran. Their second child, Cornelius Adrian (an anglicized spelling of Corey's Dutch name), had recently been born, and their second-floor apartment was getting cramped. The view looked across an unpaved street to an empty lot. The owner of the lot had already received a few offers for it, and refused them all, but she took to Corey and accepted his.

    The family masons built their third home.

    Photographs show the block walls going up, beer bottles perched on the working course, reinforcing rods sticking up, wheelbarrows, shovels and piles of sand and block, and men in undershirts smoking cigarettes.

    The ranch-style house suited the wide, shallow lot perfectly.

26   The street where Co and her family lived dead-ended at a brook.

    The street with the two new family homes on it ran off the first, and dead-ended at a pond.

    Corey and Fran's home sat in the small triangle created

by the two dead-end streets, the pond and the brook. The brook served as one of its property lines.

The neighbourhood lay in the same town and only a few blocks away from where Fran had grown up. As a child, she swam behind a mill dam a few hundred feet downstream. The mill pond served as the town's summer watering hole. The dam had been knocked over and its pond drained, but the concession booth still was standing when they moved in.

Where the one dead-end street branched from the other, a street light hung from a pole: no more than a household light bulb shaded by a tin pan. At night it cast an isolated island of illumination through the leaves, and onto the pavement directly below.

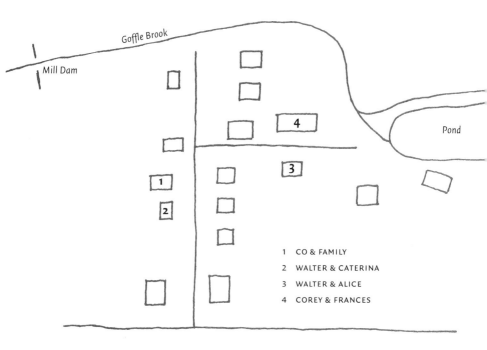

27   Corey, the electrician, installed a few non-standard electrical features in the house. Novelties.

The light switches were large, rectangular touch-plates. One of these was located in the middle of the wall above the bed in the master bedroom. It connected, not to a light, but to an outlet above the kitchen counter, into which the coffee percolator could be plugged.

A dozen and a half small, square, red push-buttons made up the switch plate in the master bedroom. If someone left a light on in the bathroom when they went to bed, or if someone was staying up too late, its red light was illumined. Push the button, the light would be extinguished.

A similar switch plate in the kitchen, with only six buttons, controlled the basement, breezeway and outdoor post-lights.

28   The upshot of all this moving and building is that Mary Ann grew up in her mother's home town, surrounded by extended family, in a setting that included a brook, pond, trees, and room to roam.

Her paternal grandparents lived across the street. Her maternal grandparents lived five blocks away.

Her aunt and uncle lived around the corner with their six children, to which they added another four. Other uncles and aunts, with more cousins, lived in nearby towns.

Mary Ann was three years old when she and her brother Neil moved into their new home. Paul and Eric were born within the next three years.

There are six people in our family; three boys, one girl and a father and a mother. We have fun together. My brothers sometimes scream and yell, but you get used to it after a while. I went to camp last summer by myself, and got homesick for my brothers' screaming. Eric used to sleep with me. At night if he was still awake when I went to bed he would throw his rubber cat at me or bang his head on the wall, then flop in his crib and start laughing. Paul, in the morning when he wakes up crabby, he will do anything like running in and out of the rooms screaming, or throwing pillows all over the house.

Neil is so slow in getting dressed. He gets up at six thirty in the morning and has to get the bus at eight fifteen, so he starts to get dressed at seven thirty and still hasn't got his shirt on at eight o'clock. It is a wonder that he has missed his bus not once yet, except when he is out of bed late.

My mother is an ordinary mother who cooks, sews, and takes care of the house and the people that live in it. My father is an electrician. Like all men he works for the money that we used to pay for the house, the car, and the truck. We used some of the money for the family, food and other things.

30 The Crawling Eye was on television every night for a week, on The Million Dollar Movie, with a matinee on Saturday. Neil and Mary Ann watched it together.

Each evening, at the point in the film when the fog came down from the Swiss mountain, hiding the horror to come, Mary Ann hid behind the television. She came out when Neil told her the scene was over.

During another scary part of the movie, Neil hid behind the television until his sister told him it was okay to come out.

He was still walking on his own at the time. On the school bus, she defended her brother from kids making fun of him falling down.

31   The familial geography began to shift.

Mary Ann's grandfather Walter died of a heart attack five years after they moved onto the street. He was fifty-nine years old. Soon after his death, Aunt Alice moved to the town where her daughter and son-in-law, Lauw, lived.

Over a short span of time, one of Corey's brothers and two of his sisters migrated to California with their families, while Co, her husband and their ten children relocated to Connecticut.

Grandma and Grandpa de Puyt still lived on Hill Street, Uncle Lauw and his wife Anne also lived relatively near, but by the time Mary Ann turned eleven years old the street had emptied of family, and for the most part so had the state.

The Duchennes, on the other hand, had moved in.

32   "Duchenne's muscular dystrophy begins insidiously, between ages 3 and 5. Initially, it affects leg and pelvic muscles, but eventually spreads to the involuntary muscles. Muscle weakness produces a waddling gait, toe-walking, and lordosis. Children with this disorder have difficulty

climbing stairs, fall down often, can't run properly, and their scapulae flare out (or "wing") when they raise their arms. Calf muscles especially become enlarged and firm. Muscle deterioration progresses rapidly, and contractures develop. Usually, these children are confined to wheelchairs by ages 9 to 12. Late in the disease, progressive weakening of cardiac muscle causes tachycardia, EKG abnormalities, and pulmonary complications."

33   No one knew, when it was built, how perfectly the single-storey ranch style design of the home would suit family needs.

All three boys stood on their own two feet for as long as they could stand on their own two feet, Eric longer than his two older brothers.

It happened by degrees. When a new house was built across the street the boys visited the construction site together. Neil rolled up to the foundation hole sitting in a wagon pulled by Eric, pushed by Paul, who was a little less free-standing and used the back of the wagon for support.

Boss and his electrical apprentice built a ramp to the front door.

34   The comedian Jerry Lewis began raising money in the 1950s for research into muscular dystrophy and to help build and maintain summer camps for "Jerry's kids" on his Labour Day shows. The shows originated in Carnegie Hall, in New York City, were later broadcast on radio, and then moved to television.

Mary Ann watched the inaugural television broadcast of the telethon on the weekend before the school year began. She was about to enter ninth grade. Seeing the parade of kids with MD, the wheelchairs, and listening to the dramatic, dire stories of the disease that Jerry told in order to solicit funds, she realized for the first time that her brothers were going to die.

35 "Prognosis varies. Duchenne's muscular dystrophy generally strikes during childhood and results in death within 10 to 15 years of onset. Death commonly results from sudden heart failure, respiratory failure, or infection."

36 *Did the boys watch the show too?*
They must have, she thinks.

37   TO THREE, BEING LOVED

You know nothing of the truth,
    the coldness
    and severity of it.
Knowing only the days of living,
    you ask not of death.
No one may deny you that.
    But even in dying,
the living
will never fade,
    because i'll remember
that you
were never waiting.

mᴠr

38   This poem, with its lower-case signature initials, lies on
     its typewritten page in one of the boxes filled with papers,
     notebooks, loose photos, photo and record albums, that we
     keep stored in the basement.
         I have made a heap of all that I could find.
         The poem dates from the poet's high-school days. There
     are more. She continued to write in college but ultimately
     abandoned the craft.
         "You wouldn't be able to handle the competition," she
     said.
         Where did she get the ability to deliver truth without
     mercy, or meanness? Medical dictionary descriptions?
         Later she said that she no longer needed to write, that it
     had served its purpose.

39   Her family home in New Jersey that we entered for the
     first time together one winter morning between our first
     and second college terms, whose threshold sent me
     sprawling, was a world unto itself, and as unremarkable as
     circumstances allowed. Neil, Paul and Eric were ten years
     past the initial diagnosis, teenagers in wheelchairs.
         Mary Ann's stories of home hadn't revealed the details
     of the daily operation of a household that revolved around
     their care, or how many people that care involved, or that
     the boys' increasing immobility mobilized ever greater
     numbers of people, or that her brothers relished each and
     every one of these messengers and ambassadors from
     the world at large, that they pounced, figuratively, on all
     newcomers.
         That there was no lack of life.

What had I expected? Bells tolling slowly. Darkness. Fear. A cowering before the inevitable.

But no one was waiting, particularly not the boys themselves.

Death did lurk, of course, especially in its minion forms such as respiratory illness. A certain vigilance maintained. Before stepping over the threshold into the breezeway, the visitor came eye to eye with a sign on the doorframe which asked them not to enter if they were unwell or communicable.

We're sitting ducks, as Eric might put it, casting a sideways look out the living room window at the ducks and geese parading along the street from the pond. The birds had lately stopped migrating, and spent the past few winters hanging about in the neighbourhood.

40 The stile says:
Please to keep you out
                            if you house a cold
or any kind of bug
                    'Cause they catch 'em with uncommon ease
            snatch 'em out of thin air
                                    field cough and sneeze
with a facility
that's second nature to physique
                            Comes
                    from being born
                                    into the game.

And you
            are in the draft

when you push the hinged door in
are one
   on the willy-nilly team
       once in
though you never really asked to join the human race now did you
but with two good legs and all parts working it should last
a lifetime and make you grateful that you don't need a hand
to lift a leg to simply piss that there but for the grace of God
go you
   in whom our obsolescence is
        what shows
who throw reflexion on
      willing and *able*
  all the livelong day
  and night
     like these three
who, to roll over in their sleep
buzzed her four times
out of bed
   and now await your sport
   in the front room.

Did you enjoy your walk, Johnny?

41 I was forever taking walks, especially during the summer
that I lived in New Jersey. With the brook running past
the house, the broken mill dam farther downstream, a
ravine, woods and windy roads, there were plenty of places
to amble. But the walks were also a pretext for escape,
a respite from the intensity and boredom. These were,

after all, nursing home conditions: bodies determinedly degenerating, time often hanging heavy, despite the activity.

There was too much time in the house. More time than anyone needed.

The irony didn't escape me: myself without direction, able to move at will; they, with a million possibilities up their sleeves, able to move only if aided.

Eric still propelled himself around the house in his wheelchair, slowly, and could lock his brakes, with some effort, when he got where he wanted, but Neil could do neither, and Paul sat the better part of the day on a chair in the living room where all three spent their time together.

Where they offered themselves to the hours.

42 You normally entered the house through the breezeway. The breezeway door opened into the kitchen, and an immediate congestion of more doorways; closet to the left, basement ahead, refrigerator to the right. This represented the one flaw in the house design. A person almost had to turn sideways to negotiate between the basement door and the fridge, and go around the kitchen table.

Skirting the table, you passed counter and sink, and above the sink a window that overlooked the front yard and the street. At that point the television came into view at the far end of the house. Walking through the dining room, veering left or right around the table, and through the front hall (with the basketball hoop hanging from the front door) brought you to the border of the boys' domain.

Neil blocked much of the open archway to the living room, seated in front of his folding card table, with his back, and the back of his chair, visible from the kitchen.

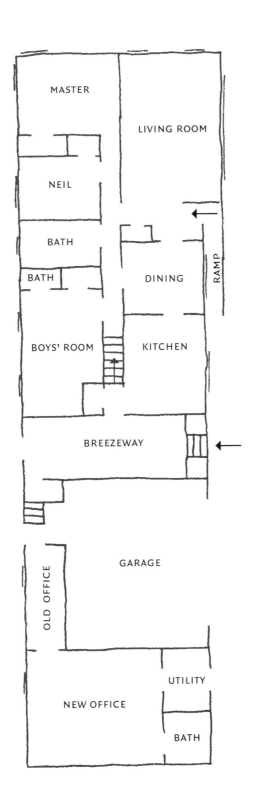

Eric sat beside him, hidden behind the wall that separated the front hallway from the living room, before his own card table. Both faced the television. A narrow corridor between their tables gave access to the room itself.

Paul's face was the first to greet you. He sat in front of Eric, positioned sideways to the television, his back to the picture window, in a living room chair. His work surface was a rickety metal TV tray.

Paul's chair placed him at an elevation where, as you entered the room, his head seemed to float on the top of Eric's table.

43   The first obligation of any visitor was to report.

The reporter had two choices. One was to remain standing at the entrance to the living room, between Neil and Eric. Boss often stood there after coming home from work. He'd lean with a left hand on the chair handle of his eldest, his right on the handle of his youngest, and shoot the breeze with his three sons.

The other choice was to walk the tight passage between their card tables and enter the circle of the room. Once within, you could sit either in the corner chair or at the far end of the couch not blocked by Neil's table.

Some preferred to remain standing, beside, and in direct competition with, the television. The television sound would be turned off during these visits, reports and encouragements from the outside world, but sometimes the picture would not, and the boys' eyes would shift irresistibly from person to screen. If the visitor stayed for any length of time they might watch TV too, or clear a spot among the piles of magazines (sports & music) and statistics sheets (sports) on Neil's table, slip between the table and the couch, and play a board game.

Visitors or friends might find themselves being mildly interrogated and simultaneously required to also adjust limbs, especially by and for Paul, who was naturally talkative and inquisitive, and as the skinniest of the three had less bulk to help keep him supported and therefore became uncomfortable more quickly.

Where did you go? (Lift my elbow onto the armrest, please)
We were there once. (Move my left foot towards the window. A little more. That's good.)

We were there once, weren't we, Otis? (Now put my arm over my head.)

We were there once, Johnny. (That's good. Thank-you.)

44   Their bodies, seated.

Neil's feet turning inward, tapering to a point, a dancer on his toes. Calves round and firm. His body mass filling the chair, with the distinctive twist at the hips that gives the torso a curve as it moves upward. A stilled *sashay*. His arms on the arm of the chair. Body leaning forward slightly, head tilted forward and to the side; neck muscles challenged by the weight of the head.

Eric and Neil share a similar physique. If Neil's bearing is regal, and it is, then Eric's may be that of the jesting monk, bent over his work, head turning to glance up at the viewer, eyes aglint.

Paul, in his chair, legs folded beneath him. Sitting like a bird in its nest. A bird *and* its nest. Shares the slim physique of his sister. In addition to the displacement and curve at the hips, there is also a more pronounced inward curve of the spine. That's his scoliosis.

The impossibility of, in particular, Paul's posture. It can't be humanly done. He sits with legs crossed, re-crossed, for hours. A yogi, twisted in meditation. Ghandi at the wheel, spinning a continuous string of words into the silence.

45   The beauty of my brothers.

46   Paul's talking, his insistent, repetitive questioning, his circling around the subject matter. He can let nothing go; the smallest detail preys on his mind, and on the ears of those around him.

Neil and Eric are reticent in comparison, though by nature Neil is at least as serious as Paul, while Eric is anything but.

Paul and Eric are referred to collectively as the boys, undifferentiated, distinct from Neil, who is closer in age to Mary Ann. Outside the family, Neil is often lumped together with them. Their shared disease gives them a single identity, although the disease itself differentiates between their body structures dramatically. They are distinct from each other, physically and in personality.

What did you expect?

I don't know. Less individuality, less liveliness.

47 "Muscular dystrophy is actually a group of congenital disorders characterized by progressive symmetric wasting of skeletal muscles without neural or sensory defects."

48 The brothers were in fact so abundant with personality that they found it necessary to divide and multiply themselves.

Otis was one of Eric's alter egos. The real Otis Taylor played professional football, in a field-position that required a physique similar to Eric's. The real Otis Taylor was not, in addition to being a football player, also an owl, but Eric's Otis was. A string of owl patio lights hung on the wall above his bed.

Eric was also Ike "behind-the-mike" White, a sports announcer, and a pig. He was not above having a little fun at his own expense.

Neil was Lamaar. He was also, and most often, Mercury Morris, another football player, the name shortened to Merkee Perkee, or just plain Merkee.

These alter egos provided the boys with more players for their team.

Paul answered to Willie. He also answered to Russell Rutherford, who was also a bull. The animal of choice may have been suggested by a play on the athlete's first name. Paul became the Bull, or Bully. In addition, he was Lenny, after the football player Lenny Dawson, who was also a seal. In his chair, his nose raised slightly, you could visualize a seal on a rock or ice floe. He was equally adept at mimicking the sound of a bull expelling air from his nose in contemplation of attack, and at barking like a seal. (Not to mention the bubbled sigh of a coffee percolator.)

They ordered pencils, embossed with their various aliases, and observed a protocol in the pencils' use. Eric kept game statistics only with his Ike White pencil.

49 Healthy, limber, young males, offering themselves up to serious play.

The athletes the boys chose were at the top of their game, used a skill, a gift, *their human bodies*, for expression.

The boys' spirits refused to be confined by their bodies' expressive limitations.

50 They lack mobility, can't walk away, or out, or take a hike; they are always displayed on the spot for who and what they are.

They have an awareness of their growing limitation of movement, and tell about it in the same way that an elderly person may relate the slow changes to their own mobility.

Eric used to be able to throw a ball, but didn't do it for a long time, he says, and now can't.

He says this as a matter of fact.

51 *Buzzed her four times / out of bed....*

Neil, Paul and Eric each had a push-button with a wire running from it that ran to the master bedroom. One of the last acts in the evening ritual of adjusting the boys' limbs into comfortable positions in bed, and in placing the pillows and soft squares of sheepskin just so, was making sure that their buzzers were placed in their grip. When they became uncomfortable during the night and wished to shift position they would buzz their mother.

Buzz their Muzzer. *Muzzer* was another of their mother's nicknames.

If they each did so only once during the night it meant that Muzzer was out of bed three times. Much like having a baby, for her. Triplets.

As their muscles went the way of their disease they became uncomfortable more quickly and more often, and the buzzing increased. A call might easily come twice or more from one or each of them. They might need more than just a limb adjusted, and it could take longer. Muzzer was moving heavy objects – her sons – incrementally, this way an inch, that way half an inch, many times, all night long.

She already ran on a minimum of sleep. Not usually free to begin her own nightly ritual of putting her hair up in pincurls before ten or eleven o'clock, she rose by six in the morning.

If it wasn't already difficult enough waking and trying to return to sleep several times a night, add to this that Boss snored.

52   The boys were largely oblivious to the amount of work they generated. Perhaps they needed to be.

Eventually they did notice their mother's mounting fatigue, and instituted an afternoon rest for her, to compensate for her nightly loss. A time during which they contracted not to bother her and she might catch some sleep. They sent her to Neil's room, where she laid on the bed to watch her favourite soap opera on the wall-mounted television.

Muzzer needed to be coaxed and needled into taking the rest, so loath was she to deprive the day of any task. The soap opera clinched it.

It was the same soap that she had listened to since it was on the radio, with the little orphan girl Mary Ann. Some of the same characters still worked the show, though not Mary Ann. Mumphy never tired of badmouthing the kindergarten teacher who, on the first day of class, abbreviated her daughter's name to Mary, after which only the family and extended family called her Mary Ann.

Back in the living room, the boys also watched the show, their eyes rolling heavenward at the implausible narrative twists, so that they could fill in any details their mother slept through.

53 The buzzing-out-of-bed woke Boss, too. He took to spending nights in his office. His old office was beside the house, behind the garage. A door off the breezeway led to a hallway behind the garage. In the hallway was a nook where the overflow fridge stood, in which the boys' fruit drinks, pop and milk, and their father's six-packs of beer, Budweiser, were kept. Three steps down from the fridge, a sliding door to the left opened into the garage, while a door straight ahead led into the office where Boss managed his electrical business.

His business went by the name Van's Electric, and Boss was known to his customers and business world in general as Van. The office was small and narrow, with room for a desk in the far corner, and in the corner by the door a closet in which he kept his work clothes.

On top of the closet sat a television. On one side of the television a small American flag hung from a pole, on the other a plexiglass frame held a coin, minted with the head of Richard Nixon on one face, an elephant on the other, and a signed note thanking him for his contribution.

A shelf beside the desk held a ham radio and weather station, from his days in the merchant marine.

Above a small cabinet decorated with switches and buttons of various kinds stood six rows of single-ounce liquor bottles, tiered like spectators standing in bleachers at a basketball game.

The bottles served as a cheering section, I hoped, when I came to request his daughter's hand in marriage.

54   By the time Mary Ann and I married, the old office was little more than an extended entrance to a self-contained apartment five times as large which had taken over the side yard.

The apartment had its own bathroom and shower. The main room had a big desk, filing cabinets, a television, an electric fireplace and a couch that pulled out into a bed.

Between the new office and the front yard was a smaller room where Boss kept a few gardening tools and a chair. Beside the chair stood an ashtray. His smoking room.

A switch controlled the light behind the plastic log-shapes in the electric fireplace. A second switch added the sound of crackling to the fire.

55   Two worlds existed within the household. The breezeway
     served as their neutral zone.
       Family life took place inside the main house, but anyone
     entering its world from the outside might not readily
     recognize in its everyday realities a connection to their own.
     They would not necessarily feel at home.
       The recognizable world existed in Boss's office.
       The geese who used to fly south now wintered by the
     pond. Their numbers had grown so large that there was talk
     of shipping them to North Carolina in transport trucks.
       The world moves beyond recognition.

56   During the winter before we were married, Neil spent six
     weeks in intensive care at the hospital.
       His apprenticeship to tubes and wires.

57   We didn't think twice about using the new office, the
     bachelor apartment, as our honeymoon suite. It suited
     Mary Ann's and my frugal taste and situation. The crackling
     fireplace added charm. The many electrical switches on the
     wall provided a variety of mood lighting.
       After the wedding and reception, bride and groom were
     chauffeured in their wedding attire to see Grandma dePuyt,
     pay respects and have photos taken. She had landed in the
     hospital with angina (Grandpa had died two years earlier),
     and was mightily displeased with herself for having to miss
     the wedding of her first grandchild to be married in New
     Jersey.
       After the visit and photograph, we repaired to Boss's
     office where a number of our college friends had already

congregated. The group came from all over, California to Chicago to Ontario. Many of us wouldn't see each other for a long time to come, since everyone had recently graduated. We drank wine, talked, opened presents and listened to records. Extended family on both sides, meanwhile, were holding their half of the wedding celebration in the house, with no idea what the young folks were up to until one of our party went to fetch more wine. Upon his return the wine-bearer related the family's surprise that the two of us were not alone.

We'll have plenty of time to be alone.

58   Mary Ann told our wedding party family stories. Her stories often seemed to involve the body, physical pratfall.

She wanted to go skating once with her friend, but the skates were in the attic. Mumphy said she would fetch them for the girls, and climbed the stairs. She was in the attic for a long time. They could hear her, rummaging. Then she called, "I can't find them. I'm coming down."

And down she came, shards of drywall following her as she broke through the ceiling and landed on the hood of the car. She had accidentally stepped between the joists. She was uninjured, though her head was bumped and slightly bleeding.

The skates landed on the hood after her.

59   Mumphy was the name more generally used around the house. A term of endearment. A two-syllable extension of Mom, that rhymed with comfy.

As other teenage boys were slowly moving away from

their mothers and fathers, these three were moving into ever greater dependence.

Muzzer gained currency when Fran began operating on automatic pilot. When the boys lost her, their mother, to the over-taxed female functionary who operated in a bit of a daze, on their behalf.

60   Boss would be in the house soon after he was buzzed, which was by 7 o'clock. Especially when the boys were still in school, it was a tightly run ship. He would come when one of them was ready to be hoisted into his wheelchair, an operation that involved Mumphy cradling their legs, under the knees, with her arms, while leaning halfway across the bed, and Boss circling his arms under the arms of his son, hands clasped together on the boy's chest.

One, two, three – they slid their son across the bed and lifted him into his chair.

"Alright, Muzzer?" he would ask. Boss usually called his wife Muzzer around the house. After each hoist he would return to the kitchen, where he drank his morning coffee while leaning over the counter looking out the window at the street, awaiting the next hoisting call. His employee would arrive, and the two would then go to work.

The *Van's Electric* truck was often parked in the driveway again by mid-afternoon. One of the perks that came with the job for Boss's single employee or apprentice was an early quitting time and the opportunity to play ball with the boys: wheelchair baseball or cap-catch on the driveway in summer; indoor hoops, floor hockey and board games in winter.

Boss, meanwhile, did business book-work in the office. He spent most of his time at home in the office, crossing the breezeway line and entering the house several times during the evening to check in, see what everyone was up to. Returning again for the hoisting back into bed. Watching television. Smoking Kools in the small utility room. Drinking Bud.

The family inside the house worried whether he was saved.

61 At least two religions existed in the family. The first was a straightforward, literalist Christianity, with an emphasis on personal salvation and piety. It originated on Mumphy's side, and involved Bible study, daily devotions and other religious activities. It came with a daily dose of television evangelists. For Mumphy, it also included the distribution of religious pamphlets to phone booths during trips to the grocery store. Grocery shopping represented a rare opportunity to witness in a tangible way, and she wasn't about to let it slip by.

"They're always gone when I come back," she'd claim, in defence of her activity to a mildly appalled daughter and son-in-law, "so someone must be taking them. I say, someone must be taking them."

The second house religion was more laissez-faire. Open-minded, non-judgmental, it allowed drinking and smoking and was tolerant, to a fault, of human failings. It stemmed from Boss's side of the family.

Concern for Boss's immortal soul went hand in hand with the distance between house and office.

62 Church was the enormous, stone-founded, wood-sided building that stood in the middle of town, almost at the top of the hill that overlooked lower Manhattan. It dated back to the wave of Dutch immigration to New Jersey in the late nineteenth century.

Mary Ann grew up going to that building. Mumphy likewise. Mumphy now usually stayed home from the morning service and listened with the boys to the broadcast over a loudspeaker hooked up to the telephone line. It allowed her to sit for a little while, though she found it difficult to resist engaging in a few small chores while the worship played in the background. Besides, if she sat still for too long she fell asleep. In the evening, after dinner, she drove to pick up her mother. Together they attended the second service.

Boss represented the family in the morning. He arrived early enough to park close to the front doors of the church, and to sit in the very back pew, under the balcony. A number of fellow early-bird regulars had seats in the same general area, and nodded to Boss and each other as they entered and sat.

When the minister's benediction released the congregation at the end of the service and the organ launched into its postlude, he was gone.

And the Lord above received no quicker message than the one Boss sent out at dinner each Sunday afternoon, and every weekday evening:

Ourfatherwhoartinheavenhallowedbethynamethykingdomcome thywillbedoneonearthasitisinheavengiveusthisdayourdailybreadand forgiveusoursinsasweforgivethosewhosinagainstusandleadusnotinto temptationbutdeliverusfromevilforthineisthekingdomandthepower andthegloryforeverandever AH MEN.

In one breath.

The first time that verbal bobsled blasted by, I felt scandalized. The prayer sounded like borderline blasphemy. And I liked to think, at the time, that I didn't have a pious bone in my body. After repeated runs, however, I couldn't help but appreciate its sheer artistry. And the breakneck speed did not, after all, disturb the universe, or the prayer's addressee.

For he was a saint, Boss was.

They all were. Are.

63   Eric is no more religiously inclined than his father, but an occasional dinner-table silence may visit him, that is almost religious.

Eric and Paul became New York Mets fans in 1969, the year the Mets unexpectedly captured the World Series. They cannot resist a victory of the underdog. It has become more than that. Eric is committed. As Neil and Paul are being pushed outdoors to engage in driveway sports on a hot summer afternoon, he chooses to stay indoors to watch the game.

"The Mets are my priority," he says.

Unfortunately, the Mets are one of those darling teams that surprise the sporting world by coming out of nowhere to win the big one, after which they fall back even more heavily into their normal, struggling ways.

"I thought we were backing a winner," says Eric.

If the Mets fail to win a game, he sinks into a funk and becomes very quiet. Neil and Boss are Yankees fans. Should the gods permit that the Yankees win on a day when the Mets lose, both Eric and Paul will ignore Boss's ribbing,

Neil's sympathetic "Maybe next time", and not speak.
Nor eat.
　Paul cannot stop talking for more than an hour.
　More disciplined, Eric enters a sulking fast that can last
for two days.

64　Mary Ann and Neil, the two oldest children, represent the
spiritual truce between their mother and father. Neither
piously moralistic nor worldly.
　With a spirit that complements both.
　A truce which circumstances have not allowed their
parents to nurture.

65　Paul is most like his mother, gravitating toward the *Are you
saved?* school. He agonizes. Agony is part of his character.
He has a cross to bear. His lack of physical bulk seems to
make him more susceptible to the winds of the psyche
which have little or no effect on his more heavily ballasted
brothers.
　He doesn't get enough protection from his linebackers.
　He thinks too much.
　A spiritual crisis claims him in earnest when he
concludes that he is not living up to the requirements
placed upon a believer, the requirement to spread the word,
that the television evangelists have been happily driving
home over the airwaves, wagging their fingers at the
camera.
　OurFatherwhoartinheaven...
　Can I get a witness?

Can we see by 40 watts
With groping hope
and coffee pots:
Our wager with the ancient sages,
To grip their scope
in five short pages?
      The shadows of illumined dials,
A humming clock to pace the style
And space apart the growing pile
Of books that blur
And those still open:
The dots connect with bighand motion.

Oh, to see beyond this time
With penitence enough to rhyme.

mυr

67   After the wedding, Boss drove us, with our limited worldly
possessions, in the van that had been specially outfitted for
the boys – removable seats, floor-straps to keep their chairs
from rolling, an aluminum ramp, and an air conditioner
that sat on top of the van's roof like a flat-topped cupola.
We were bound for our new home in Toronto.
      At the border crossing we were pulled aside and escorted
into a small room. There, a man behind a desk questioned,
scolded, threatened and generally threw his official weight
around, until he finally succeeded in making a twenty-one

year-old woman cry. In the midst of writing papers and exams during her last months before graduating from college, Mary Ann had also managed to chase down and fill out all the paperwork required in order to enter Canada as a landed immigrant, but between moving from one location to the other, her visa hadn't caught up with her before we left New Jersey.

At her tears, the official relented a little, and said that the only way he could allow her into the country was if she received special, ministerial permission. The only way to obtain that permission was from the minister himself, in Ottawa. Our new friend then picked up the telephone and dialled.

The minister was hosting a barbeque. Mary Ann's fate hung on how well the meat on the grill was cooking. It must have been perfect. Permission was bestowed, in triplicate.

We walked out of the building into the daylight, feeling seared.

Boss's arm rested on the open window of the van, a cigarette in his fingers. He was talking, sharing a laugh with one of the guards.

68 Hello Brother in Law John and Mary Ann, not Mary as you would say John ARE YOU GETTING INTO A RUT YET OR IS THE ROUTINE CLOSING IN? John Your hampering your education by going to college if there are colleges in Canada. Guess who my favorite teacher was in school? (Ed Ucation of course) Just a little joke. Mary Ann are you giving John a lot of stereo dinners? you cant have TV dinners

because you don't have a TVThis is a thesis compared
tosome of my other letters in my carreer 82 words

> Sincerely,
> your soul brother
> OTIS

69   Eric's proudest moment came when he dropped out of high
school. This set him apart from his brothers, placed him
outside of the social norm, and gave him bragging rights.

He liked to remind me that his sister's real name, her
family name, was Mary Ann. I had fallen into step with her
kindergarten teacher and the rest of the world outside the
family in calling her Mary.

Neither Eric nor Paul had the muscle-power any longer
to strike the keys of a manual typewriter, and handwriting a
letter would have been too labourious, so they had put their
money together to buy an electric typewriter, and launched
their writing career. A career that consisted mostly of letters
northbound.

Paul appended his words to the bottom of the same sheet
of paper that Eric had started:

70   Dear Brother In-Law John and Sister Mary Ann

Have jobs yet? if you do I hope your doing good.Eric(Otis)
suggests that you hire a butler when you can afford itto take
care of your house during the day while your keeping your
nose to the grindstone.

Mary Ann do you miss the trees,birds,chipmunks,squirr
els,and the quietness.and how does it feel to be the boss of
the household?

John do you miss playing games and throwing tennis balls at our gloves?Now we are asking the exercise ladies to play games with us when they are done with the exercises.

We have been playing the wedding to all the exercise ladies and they all liked it because it was simple and their was nothing put on.Eric(Otis)was sick of hearing it and was threatening to erase the tape but I think he was only joking.

Did you like Reverend Wisse's baseball joke?Neil(Mercury) asked him to do it.Eric(Otis)said it was the highlight of the reception.We are going to invite Reverend Wisse and two of his boys with us to a baseball game Friday night June 28.

Tuesday Dennis and Kevin were cutting Hoag's grass and found three cute little bunny rabbits without their mother.The next day their cat Mittens killed them that mean cat.Well I guess thats their nature.

When John graduates from college and when you buy your house or estate you should write a thesis on trying to get into Canada without a Visa and starting a living without furniture,a stove,and a refrigerator.

It gives me great pleasure to write to you for the first time,

Your Brother and Brother In-law,

PAUL

71   Eric's threat to erase our wedding tape came in the context of the Watergate trials, which dominated the airwaves at the time.

We shared a house with another couple. Laura had been a friend of Mary Ann's since second grade. Together and separately the four of us travelled back and forth to visit New Jersey several times; as often as we had the time and felt the family urge. But we were embarking on our own lives, and Mary Ann's parents never once made us feel as though we had a duty to anything but our own independence.

From very early on Mary Ann had been given what first struck me as a surprising degree of independence. The household, and her parents' attention, naturally focussed itself on her three younger brothers, and left her, the eldest, free. It was as though Fran and Corey did not want their daughter to be drawn into the vortex of care, and preferred to have one person in the family who could prove that what had happened to their family was not the final word. To show the world that everyday normalcy still existed after diagnosis. An ambassador child.

In effect, Mary Ann was left to raise herself; the sweet-voiced orphan girl from the radio show. And she possessed the gift to do so.

72 After three years we'd had enough of the big city and wanted to move closer to my family, who were are all living an hour to the west.

Before relocating, we decided to travel.

We purchased a Volkswagen van, vehicle of choice for the quasi-hippie traveller, and outfitted its interior as a camper by employing Mary Ann's advanced skills as seamstress, and my more rudimentary skills as a carpenter. Our possessions were stored in my parent's basement, and we set off on a footloose, year-long journey across and around the North American continent. It was early September.

At a gas stop in a small town, the van wouldn't start. Its

electrical system seemed to have a direct connection to our unexpressed anxieties.

We spent our first overnight in a campground on Lake Huron, a serene setting among sand dunes and trees. Our fellow campers were the non-summer people; travellers, retirees. We lay in the back of the van, listening to the sound of a violin being played quietly into the cooling air, and were soothed.

Second stop, Grand Rapids, Michigan, where Mary Ann's Uncle John, Fran's older brother, introduced us as his "retired niece and her husband." He was perplexed and bemused by our plan. We were both twenty-four years old.

Then stops in various cities to visit far-flung friends from college days, friends who were getting on with their lives just as we seemed to be taking leave of ours. Our last planned visit was to be New Jersey, from where we would officially launch the transcontinental tour. We were thinking Florida Keys for the winter. We drove up and down the vividly coloured mountains of Pennsylvania, in driving rain, barrelling through the evening without a break, afraid to hazard a stop because the van was again acting up, and coasted into Mary Ann's driveway sometime after midnight.

73 DECEMBER 19

Dear Frank and Martha,

Glad to hear from you. We've been so immersed in the activities of this household for so long, with little contact with the outside "normal" world, we're a bit surprised each time we receive a letter that life, indeed, does exist in other forms.

We've put 60 miles on our VW since we came here in late
September. The availability (and 8 cyl. guts) of my parents'
Nova, the inconsistency and ailing trans. of our van and
the withering of our wanderlust have kept us parked for
some time. Our "journey" *has* continued, however, though
perhaps would be classified as one of a more spiritual
sort than one measured on our rather neglected Rand
McNally's. Being in a home where Death continually haunts
the doorways, held at bay by God's most valiant Angels,
certainly puts life on a different plane. And being in close
contact with angels is an experience hard to part with....

love, Mary

74   What we found when we arrived was a ratcheting-up in
what it took to care for Mary Ann's brothers. The household
was being overwhelmed by these demands, and by
something else; something less tangible was in the air.

The routines of the house remained as predictable
and uneventful, for the most part, as ever, if also more
intense. Cars lined the curbless street, to transport the
people who were coming and going to work, visit, or
volunteer. A licensed practical nurse was on duty seven
days a week, eight hours a day; a second LPN came in the
evening. A homemaker (from an agency) came five days,
for eight hours a day. Volunteers came in the morning,
daily, to exercise the boys, and in the evening to help feed
Neil. Friends and neighbours dropped by to visit or bring
something. A deaconess from the church came once a week
to do "mending, ironing, folding laundry, etc." Twice each
week the deaconesses brought dinner to the house.

75 Mumphy made a list of all their names, later, when she had the time, on the backs of the discarded envelopes and advertising flyers that accumulated in the kitchen, between the toaster and a pencil cup.

The list included eight LPNs, five homemakers, and twenty "exercise ladies," as the boys called the women who came to help them move their limbs. The woman who brought audio tapes and sports magazines each week. The neighbour who saved the newspapers and *Sporting News* that lay stacked on the stairs down to the basement.

Much of the weekday traffic to the house was female, but on the back of another envelope Mumphy listed twelve of the boys' friends, ones who regularly visited after the boys became homebound. Dennis, from across the street, came almost daily. Jay, who was Boss's employee and just a year older than Neil. A couple of men came in the evening to help with feeding Neil. The church minister often stopped by for a few minutes.

Johnny Vander Meer, a hometown boy and baseball pitcher from the 1950s whose fame lay in pitching two no-hitters in a row for Boston, came by and signed a couple of baseballs for the boys. He had his photo taken with them for the newspaper.

76 No one from the outside world might have known or discovered what was going on in the home, or what help was needed, if Mumphy hadn't left it briefly, hadn't travelled on a vacation, a respite, to California, to visit her sister. A neighbour offered to provide daily care for the boys. Before she left, Mumphy said to the neighbour, who was a registered nurse, "Don't you let any of my boys end up in the hospital."

If one of the boys ended up in the hospital it would mean that their care was too much for one person, which would mean that they had already entered a territory outside her power to regulate or control. It would mean exposure and, ultimately, grief.

The neighbour quickly discovered the amount of work involved. One of the boys did have a crisis. He did not end up in hospital, but the family situation was laid bare to the minister and church, and by the time of Mumphy's return an LPN was in place, a homemaker soon after.

77 Mary Ann and I entered into the fabric of the routines, the comings and goings. It was quieter in the house than perhaps it sounds: more like life on ward than in emergency room. The loudest intrusions into the silence were produced by a portable machine used for Paul and Eric's "treatment", and Neil's suctioning machine. Both were intermittent and relatively brief. There was the television, too, but not always, and never loud. Occasionally Paul, a.k.a. the Bull, would bellow, or call out "Helloooo Merkeeeee" to Neil in his bedroom. To which Merkee would reply with a Morse code of blasts from his buzzer. Neil's card table in the living room remained in place should he wish to make a cameo appearance, but by then he spent all of his time in bed.

The constant was the tall-treed quiet of a dead-end street running off a dead-end street. It was more peaceful than it ought to have been with three boys in their late-teens and early-twenties, for at the heart of all the day-to-day movement and activity lay the deepening stillness of their three bodies.

78 That the activity seemed to be reaching a climax was the intangible something else.

It hadn't gone unnoticed, this intensifying. The slow, years-long buildup had been a form of preparation, but when you place its slowness beside what it was building up to, you can see where a blindness might have developed, an unconscious refusal to admit that what was happening was actually happening, or where it all was leading.

Denial as positive force.

No one knew for sure what would happen, or how, or when, so why waste time and energy on conjecture?

And no one likes to think they're working for a hopeless cause.

79 With its nurses in uniform, hospital beds, hydraulic hoist, and the whiff of ammonia, home had indeed taken on the atmosphere of a hospital. At the same time, the hospital itself had become almost as familiar as home. Grandma de Puyt had been admitted more than once, Eric had done a short stint and Paul had spent a few days there earlier in the spring. But Neil was the family's hospital pro. He'd endured his first, six-week stay during the months before we were married, and spent another six weeks there while we were living in Toronto.

His sister and I visited his bedside between college terms during his first, long sojourn in Intensive Care. This was new territory for everyone in the family, and a time of great, silent suffering.

A tracheotomy was performed then, to relieve the pressure on his respiratory system and make it easier to suction the fluid from his lungs.

STRANGLE HOLDS

You stubborn Dutchman!
It's your grip that shames me,
The way you skip rope in your sleep
Those plastic tubes your private game of double dutch.

Smack your lips in agile pride
That tube was dinner in disguise.

You damn hollander!
Can't you ever sit one out?

If just this time
I'd rip your rope,
trip you up,
teach you virtue in sitting–

I can't,
brother.

it's time for me to wait my turn
when strangle holds
have held back death.

mur

81 Neil's condition in the hospital deteriorated during that
stay, but no one in the family knew how critical it had
become, until later. As the bills from those six weeks
accumulated on the kitchen table and Mumphy negotiated
her way through the confusing levels and hallways of the
family's medical insurance policies, she learned, almost as
an aside, that at a critical point during his stay the doctors
who reviewed hospital cases had taken a vote on whether or
not to pull the plugs on the machines that were doing Neil's
breathing for him.

There were five doctors.

Two voted to pull. Two, not.

The family doctor had cast the deciding vote.

82 That Neil got better seemed a miracle, that he was able to
return home, a gift. That he lived, grace.

Merkee the returning hero, bearing the scars from the
journey, the frontiers this disease had taken him to. Holy
lands it might take his two younger brothers to as well.

Neil did not regale brothers, sister or parents with tales
around the family campfire, under the stars. The story was
his body, and his body sufficed.

83 After his tracheotomy (that gauze necklace with its plastic opening and rubber bauble centred on his throat; his medal from the war), suctioning Neil's lungs became one of the daily household tasks. It was usually conducted by the practical nurse, but Mumphy learned the procedure as well. The rubber cork removed from its hole allowed a plastic tube to be fed down Neil's throat and into his lungs. A pump humming on the bedside table created the vacuum that suctioned up the accumulated fluid. Suctioning was both routine and extraordinary, and it could hurt. He winced as the tube went down. It was painful simply to watch.

Not long after our arrival Mary Ann had entered into the evening care routines with her brothers. Now she learned the suctioning procedure as well, so as to be able to fill a back-up role in case of emergency, and as a sisterly act.

They like to be touched, she said.

Meaning that her brothers liked to be handled in ways and for reasons that were not solely functional but also affectionate, familiar, human. She made sure that she gave them that touch, in hugs and kisses, with her hands when she spread the cream and ointments over their bodies. Suctioning the brother closest to her in age and temperament was not exactly what she had in mind, but had been given nonetheless.

84 They are touched and handled often, of course. Creams and ointments line the shelves.

Eric had a cold. Mumphy spread a vaporizing rub for congestion over his chest, working it well into his skin, as he was sitting up in bed.

Within a few minutes his face began to turn noticeably red. Then it grew to a deeper red, an almost fiery red. It wasn't the furnace thermostat gone haywire, but Mumphy having picked up the wrong plastic tube. She'd rubbed a liniment for sore muscles into his chest.

85 Eric's a good sport. All evening, the sweat pouring down his face.
  "I'm steamed," he says.
  Mumphy has too much on her mind.

86 Eric likes to be physical. He wants to wrestle. I tuck my head under his arm (him sitting in his wheelchair) and he puts me in a full nelson, with sound effects. His muscles are so lax. He puts all his strength into the most tender, gentle of wrestling holds.
  He throws his head back and bops me on the back, when I fool on the piano behind him.
  His arm lies on his card table, he looks sideways over at me sitting on the couch, and snaps his fingers, the long delicate thumb and middle finger riding against each other silently. I provide the audio with these same fingers that tap the lettered keys.

87 Their bodies going in two directions at once.
  Their bodies growing up and growing backward, at the same time.
  Why they will remind you, with the delicacy of their

hands, the softness of skin, their muscle tone, why they will remind you of an infant.

Why my daughter's arm on her highchair will remind me of her uncle's arm on the arm of his wheelchair; will remind me that in order to grow, a body needs to be *able* to grow.

To grow, a body needs to grow.

Why, at nineteen years, the child in Eric is alive, his body going.

88 The exercise ladies are women from the community, the church community most of them. Some have children, and might bring a preschool-aged child along. Others have grown children and are now volunteering. They are given training in the stretches that help keep the boys limber. It is not a complicated task.

The lady of the day enters the living room and kneels in front of Paul, who is seated in his chair, and takes his hand in one of her own hands. The two are at eye level. She massages and flexes his fingers individually. She takes his elbow in her other hand, and gently bends and unbends his arm; one arm, then the other. She unfolds his legs and does the same for them. These exercises are simple, and similar for each of the boys, although their different physiques mean that attention is concentrated in different bodily locations. Paul likes to have his arm placed up and behind his head and left there for a few minutes. Eric can still do this for himself.

The women do for the boys what the boys can no longer do themselves, are providing them with muscle.

Boss used to do these small exercises with them when

they were younger, when it didn't take as long, and didn't have to be done every day. And when it did not cause him so much personal grief.

As the ladies work, kneeling before the stationary young men, they talk. They answer questions, in Paul's case, and offer conversation. Or they offer silence. Some are more naturally voluble than others, or have a more readily sparked sense of humour. Every one of them has a sense of humour. Good humour is the common currency of the household and its serving community.

The conversational music ebbs and flows, the limbs bend and stretch; a seated, slow motion dance, the lady leading.

89   When the morning exercises end, the games begin. Games are a part of the daily routine, and participation is included in the job description of every volunteer and most visitors who stay longer than five minutes.

Probe. Dominos. Sorry. Longhorn. Fang Tang. Scrabble. Crazy Eights. Rack-O. Yahtzee. Strato-matic. Aggravation. Gotcha. Chinese Checkers. Obsession. Mousetrap. Parcheesi. Concentration. War. Go for Broke. Billionaire. Othello. The Game of Life. Monopoly.

The closet in Paul and Eric's bedroom, then in Neil's bedroom, and finally in Mary Ann's bedroom in the basement, and under her bed, grows stacked with boxes of boards, player pieces, dice, marbles and cards.

90   The exercise lady of the day is often asked to pen an entry into Paul's diary:

"When I arrived I was greeted by two cow bells, then I had a keep fit lesson with Neil as he had me dashing about catching ping pong balls."

"Well I've just arrived and before I start I think I'll go and join Eric who is in the best place of all: bed. However, with these two slave drivers waiting for me I had better wake up and get going."

"I won! I won! I won! Finally after months of defeats I finally won a game. The score for the record was, Me 270, Paul 230, Eric 155 and Neil 40. What a nice way to start the day. See you next Thursday."

91   Eric keeps lists and statistics on the exercise lady's volunteer visits, the games played, the wins and losses. His graduate degree is in gamesmanship, with a minor in statistics. His truncated high school career has not inhibited a pursuit of knowledge, it merely capped-off a relationship to the institution that had been strained since third grade. At sixteen, he wanted to exercise some control over his destiny.

Paul has gone through all twelve grades. As has Neil, the wave-breaker. Neil took his education as far as he could, attending a semester in business studies at a community college, before his first extended hospital stay prevented returning for a second semester. He is less naive than his younger brothers and has a web of friends that extends farther from the house. Being in a wheelchair, needing help, meant that he met people.

The high school at first refused to grant Neil a diploma. He lacked a single required credit in on-the-road driving instruction.

92 No diploma gives Eric an excuse. If he loses a game, it's because he's a high school dropout; if he wins, the headline reads, "College Bum Drops One To High School Dropout." His second minor degree is in one-liners.

After a knock-out move in Scrabble, in which the college bum moved from a dead-last scoring position to winner by setting down a word that employed all seven letters, landed on two triple-word scores, and emptied the letter bin, thereby ending the game and giving him additional points from the leftover letters on his competitors' racks, Eric said:

"Looks like Johnny's turning pro."

The Bull lowers his head, and bellows.

93 Mary Ann and I often sleep in.

It's noted in the diary that Paul keeps; or between the lines. Not that there is much room between Paul's lines. His diary pages are narrow-lined paper, three inches wide by six inches high, which can be removed from and snapped into a six-ring, memo binder. They are the perfect size for him to use on his TV tray table, resting his wrist against the table's edge, his fingers gripping the pen, moving a fine spidery script across the small page, chronicling the day in its web.

TUESDAY
Oct.25 1. Got treatment at 9:25
2. 9:00 John T. got me out of bed 3. Emma came at 7:45 4. Emma started working me at 8:15 because Neil had to be suctioned a lot 5. M.A. got out of bed

by 12:50 6. Mrs. Floyd came at 11:20
and left by 12:20 7. John played piano
at 12:50 8. Mumphy layed down at
1:14 9. John finished playing the piano
at 1:22 10. 1:50 to 2:10 M.A. trimmed John's
beautiful locks of hair 11. Had my treatment from 2:05 to 2:35. I had it longer
because of extra phlegm 12. Emma left
at 2:35.

What the scribe generously leaves out is that John T. likely
returned to bed after lifting Paul out of his. Mary Ann and I
are afforded the opportunity to sleep off the exhaustion that
the house produces, a luxury not available to Mumphy.

We're emotionally overwhelmed by what's going on here,
though only dimly aware of that fact.

M.A. is Mary Ann in his diary. Emma is the LPN who
comes each day, and Mrs. Floyd the nurse who comes
weekly to check up on the home situation and determine
when, for instance, Neil will need to have his tracheotomy
changed. The "treatment" Paul is receiving is a kind
of mechanical inhaler. It is becoming more and more
important as a way of breaking up the liquid and phlegm
that accumulates in his and Eric's lungs. Which they
then spit up into a special bowl. Sputum is a word in their
vocabulary. Neil is suctioned for the same reason.

Paul takes very seriously the aspects of his health care
that he has some control over. He enters the sound of
the machine rumbling on the TV tray beside him, while
concentrating on breathing through the mask. He
complains that Neil's television in the bedroom down the
hallway distracts him.

94   We sleep in the basement, where it is pitch black, in the bedroom that Boss built for Mary Ann when she entered junior high school. Until then she had shared a room with Eric, the one that now is Neil's. Her basement room has remained unchanged since her high school days, except for the infiltration of board games: wood panelling on the walls, acoustic tile on the ceiling; white, French Provincial (more or less) dresser, desk and shelving units.

The room's novel electrical feature is the heating panel in the ceiling.

The wood panelling was removed once, after Mumphy accidentally dropped her wedding ring behind the kitchen counter. Boss took apart the cabinets upstairs, in search, couldn't find it and concluded that the ring must have fallen farther down, and so took Mary Ann's panelling off her bedroom wall.

Still missing, the ring rests somewhere in the wall behind our heads as we sleep.

95   We like it here.

We are grace notes to family life. We pick up the slack. We perform errands and do chores around the house. Mary Ann sews; I fix things. She is engaged in a kind of brother-care that she never did as a teenager, mostly because this care was not necessary then. She has crossed over into another territory as sister and caregiver.

Together we assemble a family photo gallery on the wall in the dining room. We rake the leaves at Grandma's house and put up her storm windows. We are arms and legs, youth and vigour (except for sleeping in).

Is this not purpose?
It will soon be winter.

96   We come as help and witness.

97   We were sitting in the kitchen with Mumphy when she
     asked if Mary and I could stay on longer than we'd planned.
     She said that she and Boss had talked about it. We intended
     to leave by the end of October, but that date was quickly
     approaching and our plans for travel had begun to feel very
     disconnected and abstract. Or we became disconnected
     from the plans.
         They had never asked such a thing before.
         We said yes.
         The family back in Ontario didn't quite know what to
     make of the decision, at first. To them it seemed Mary Ann
     and I were giving up on adventure, putting off the future,
     and to what end? They didn't understand the situation.
         No one can understand, unless they're in it. We were in it
     and we hardly understood ourselves.
         Even if you see it coming, you cannot see it coming.

98   It is not our life.
         This is what makes it possible to say yes to staying. Our
     life ended when we packed up and left Toronto, and the
     next life has not yet begun. We are living in-between.
         We participate. We are not the principals.
         We are grateful that this life is not ours.

99   We began the outdoor adventures by rolling Paul and Eric through the neighbourhood to attend a fall fair held in the church parking lot, wheeling among the booths and tables, eating hot dogs.

Later in the month we dressed the two boys and ourselves up for Halloween and went trick-or-treating. Paul wore a brown cape, with a cowbell around his neck. People often presented him with bull-paraphernalia. His head was adorned with two horns, and the sign propped against his chest said, "Beware of Bull." Mary Ann pushed his chair, wearing a t-shirt with a bull's head displayed on it and the words "Property of Chicago Bulls."

Eric wore a green, numbered jersey. He had dark smudges rubbed under his eyes, a peewee football sitting next to him in the chair and a helmet gripped by the face guard in his hand. He adopted the appropriately fearsome look of a linebacker. I was his referee; black sweater, with a whistle around my neck.

We spent the late afternoon going door to door in the neighbourhood. There is true shock value, we discovered, an authentic Halloween scare, in rolling two young men with unusually disposed bodies to someone's front door, even if the two are known to the neighbour whose door is being knocked upon.

People didn't know how to respond. We laughed and horsed around in the face of what they perceived as a kind of physical horror.

When Mary first began telling me stories about her brothers, I was secretly appalled at her lightness of tone in relating things so patently serious, and the same principle must have been at work among the neighbours. When you live at the working, everyday end of disability or disease

you tend not to show as much respect for its limitations
as others feel it is only proper to show. It leaves others at a
disadvantage.

You can't help but feel a bit sorry for them.

100   I bumped into Beer Belly Bob while out for a walk in the
morning.

Bob got his name from Paul once when the boys saw him
coming home with a case of beer.

He was raking leaves, and leaning on his rake, talking
to his sister. Bob and Frieda live across from each other,
around the corner, where they have lived since before
Boss's parents and sister moved onto the street.

They were standing together at the corner, where a patch
of tall bamboo grows.

Two sentences into our conversation, as though he had
long been waiting to tell this to someone on the inside, Bob
said:

"It's a real shame about those boys."

I was stunned. How could he say such a thing? Is it
true? Shame had never occurred to me, and it made me
feel disloyal, simply hearing the word said. If I nodded
agreement, would that not somehow diminish who my
brothers are?

And they are grand.

101   In an effort to find more comfortable seating for Eric, Mary
Ann and I looked around in second-hand furniture stores
until we found a chair we thought could be modified for his
needs. She sewed a seat and back pillow, while I worked to

make the chair's arms removable, give it a back that could be adjusted to various angles, and put it on wheels.

We spent the next few days, a week, two weeks, trying out the new chair with him, moving his arms and legs a little this way, that way, placing the small pieces of soft sheepskin where it seemed they might do the most good; all to no avail. Eric didn't want to disappoint, but there wasn't much that could be done about his discomfort.

The chair sat empty in the corner of the living room for a time afterward.

"It's not that I don't like your chair," he said. "You know, the spirit is willing but the flesh is weak."

102   One Saturday we pushed Paul to church, about five blocks away. The big stone and clapboard building was open. We toured around inside, and he played one-fingered organ. He hadn't set foot, or rolled, into church, or attended a service, in quite a while. Not for ten years, in fact. He and Eric worked it out later: it happened before this, and after that. They batted events back and forth until the chronological slot was filled.

They turn events over and over again in their conversation, like jewels. The cut is always the same but the light it refracts may change.

As we toured, Paul wondered if he could come again the next morning.

103   He loved it.

From the parking lot, the accessible doors of the building opened into the very front of the church, beside the pulpit,

so no one could miss us the next morning as we entered
and rolled the length of the filled sanctuary to where Boss
was sitting in his usual place in the back row. Paul had
a bird's-eye view of the pulpit down the centre aisle. He
croaked quietly along with the singing, clearly savouring
each note, every minute.

While the congregation was standing for the final hymn,
we rolled down the centre aisle to the doors we'd come
in through, and found a small room behind the pulpit
where Paul could use the urinal. He sat with the plastic
blue container between his legs during the minister's
benediction and as the organ pipes, which were housed
in the same room, blasted us with the opening chords of
the postlude. Then we returned through the doors to the
parking lot, where many people came by to say hello, and
how glad they were to see him there.

Eric wanted to get in on the action, so the next morning
we wheeled the two of them to the church again, and gave
him the tour. They signed the guest book.

104 And as we sport with Paul and Eric, Neil keeps quiet daily
vigil in his room, attended day and evening by his nurses.

105 Eric's birthday.
A visitor to the house tonight told us that they're
thinking of keeping their daughter out of the college they
had previously selected for her, because the college is now
teaching dance to its students.

"When you see the way a man and a woman dance

together sometimes, well, it's nothing but a sin," the visitor said.

We were in the living room at the time of this conversation, Paul and the birthday boy in attendance.

Lying in bed, still upset, Mary Ann found the words that hadn't come a few hours earlier: "Don't you think the one thing my brothers would like to do is get up and *dance?*"

106 Paul and Eric have invented a night game.

During their preparations for bed, they hatch and develop the concept, and then enlist their mother and sister to do the work, to place a source of illumination in an unusual setting.

That is how the plastic pumpkin, with a small candle burning within it, came to be floating in the toilet bowl of their small bedroom washroom. It is also how the bedsheet came to be spread across the room, creating a tent-like effect under which a flashlight burned within a ring of stones.

When the light is in location, the overhead light (a basketball poised halfway through its hoop) is doused, and they call in their brother-in-law. He assesses their creation for inventiveness and humour, compares it to their previous efforts, and awards them points on a scale from one to ten.

His point system is subjective and open to abuse. They accept or argue their score.

Johnny's getting hard to please in his old age.

They suggest a sleepover. When they were younger they took turns sleeping in a tent in the backyard with their sister. The same flannel sleeping bag used then is unrolled onto the linoleum floor, next to the flashlight, under the spread sheet.

107 It is getting sadder, here.

Both boys take much longer to get set in a comfortable position, and last for shorter periods.

Mornings, Paul is washed, dressed in bed, and wheeled into the living room before Eric, partly because he is lighter in weight and easier to handle, partly because of the amount of time needed to seat Eric comfortably after he has been hoisted into his chair. It is now possible to spend more than an hour, two hours, with the minute adjustments and readjustments to the position of his body and limbs.

They know how frustrating it is for their mother and sometimes, especially Paul, would rather be uncomfortable than bother her any more than they have already.

Eric now enters the living room often later than mid-morning.

Or, as Paul notes in his diary: "E. rolled in L.R. at 10:31," "E. checked in L.R. at 11:10," "E. zipped in," "made the scene," "barrelled," "E. bombarded into living room at 10:50," "sneaked," "made himself known," "brightened up the living room," "scampered," "barged in," "bombarded," "zoomed"....

In his entries Paul never refers to his alter-ego-rich brother as Otis or Ike, but always by his Christian name. The difficulties test Eric's humour, and Mumphy's patient endurance. He does not want to spend so much time dealing with his body. It takes away from his other, more pressing activities. His scribe-work.

108 As researchers delve ever more deeply into the disease, like scholars to a text, trying to discern how the Word, in this instance, is made flesh....

This is the bad Word. This is the Word you don't want to hear, that is rarely spoken of from the pulpit.

For there will be disease, and it will take many forms.

It will strike high and low.

And it will ravage the body; the body personal, the body familial.

109 Is it an invasion of Neil's privacy to speak of his tears?

His mother was dressed and ready to pick up Grandma for church when he requested the bedpan. Again. For a third time in two hours. With equally unsuccessful results.

Here, you hardly know what privacy is.

110 Boss and Mumphy were asked to attend a council meeting with the elders and deacons of the church, and Mary Ann and I were invited as family members to come with them. The church had been helping out the family in a major financial way, funding the hiring of the LPN and homemaker, and they wanted to talk about the situation in the house.

We didn't know what to expect. The men in the room seemed a bit officious.

"As called by this local church to be stewards, we seek the best way to fulfill our call."

Perhaps they were frightened by what they were about

to suggest. They asked about the boys and home life in general, and then the conversation turned to the question of whether it would be desirable, for all concerned, if one or more of the boys were to enter a long-term care facility.

The elders had the right, and an obligation, to bring this up with the family. They were concerned with the state of everyone's health, especially Fran's, as well as the church budget. The cost, especially to her, of caring for the boys, was visible. That cost, as well as the home-care costs, could only increase. We were all aware of that.

"Try not to look at this as abandoning your children, but as doing the best for them and for yourself."

We listened, knowing the whole time that they could talk until the cows, the bulls, the owls and the seals came home, but the family would not need to consider or confer for one moment, because the idea of sending the boys away was a non-starter.

To the elders' credit they respected and accepted a simple no without argument. It seemed as though they had anticipated what the answer would be.

111   I went to sit with Neil in his room when we got home. He knew what was up. I told him about the meeting and the elders' suggestion. This veteran of intensive care, two extended hospital stays and medical interventions, and of suffering, looked at me and asked, "Who'd be the first to go?"

He was smiling. He knew the answer.

One Saturday night, the four of us went to visit Aunt Alice and Uncle John for dinner. The idea was to foster a bit of a social life for Boss and Mumphy. They had none, together or apart.

Aunt Alice had married into the Boss's family twice, while outliving, thus far, three husbands. Her first husband abandoned her with four children. Her second husband was Boss's father, Walter. When Walter died, she married a man who had multiple sclerosis. She nursed him until he died, then married Walter's brother, John. Her marriage to John was the one that had been made for them in heaven, given late in life. The couple were obviously happy, and a going concern. They'd kept Mary Ann and me up into the wee hours more than once, when we came to visit. We wanted to be like them when we got old.

Aunt Alice was the mother of Ann, who was the wife of Boss's brother, Lauw. Ann and Lauw also joined the evening.

This is Mumphy, then, entering into a situation where she is meant to be Fran again; a social situation. Boss has no difficulty, is in his element. He is familiar with operating on this level; he does so on a daily basis with his customers. Everyone else is equally at ease, engaged. Our bodies are relaxed.

Fran sits, either with a glazed look on her face or in constant motion, pulling up a sock, picking at a piece of invisible lint, not able to enter the circle of conversation.

We have dinner and afterwards the men head down into the basement to play pool. It's simple to be normal, to act as a functioning human being.

She is overtaxed, has no alternate.

She works eighteen-hour days nursing her three sons,
who are diminishing under her hands.

She cannot turn off, cannot readjust her focus.

She seems no longer fit for this world, a world which the
rest of us are at pains to enjoy.

113 In order to pursue a conversation with Mumphy, one has to
pursue her through the house, one room to the other, one
chore to the next. It's an effort to keep up.

There is an element of the frantic in her motion.

She asks, lately, "How long can I keep it up? What do I
pray for?"

This is new.

114 Boss often gets impatient with Mumphy because of her
constant activity during dinners at home. She sits, she
stands, she gets this, that, she gets nothing. It makes for
tense times around the table, which is almost the only time
they spend together.

We showed slides of Mary Ann's and my truncated, transcontinental journey, and in the process of setting up for the
show discovered a box of slides from Boss and Mumphy's
honeymoon travels, another box with the first years of
their marriage, when Mary Ann was born, and more of the
building of the house.

They settled into a surprising ease with each other on
the couch, bantering dates and places between them as
amiably and lightly as Eric and Paul might, determining
the provenance of the images on the wall, where they were

on that day, what they'd done there, helping each other out with the details.

We were allowed a brief glimpse into their attraction to each other as a young couple, as Fran and Corey, visiting from a time put out of mind, adjusting the limbs of their marriage into a more comfortable position, one where their bodies still touched.

115   He has no wife.

He is an outsider in his own house. His only companion in the family was Mary Ann, who is now taken.

Uncle John says, "It's hard on him to have three kids laid up. He can't have a normal home life."

I think, *Who* cannot have a normal home life?

116   I sit in the breezeway during the evenings when I want to be alone, in the neutral zone between office and house. Boss passes through several times to see what's up in the house.

I am free to drink his beer. Which I drink freely. It is stocked in the beverage fridge. This is not the source of the tension between us. The boys have taken to calling me, among other designations, "the father-figure," in playful reference to my presence in the house and to the hoisting chores I've taken up, partly because of Boss's bad back, largely because I am there and don't have to be buzzed.

The reference is also to their father's increasing absence in the house, which is partly due to my doing the hoisting chores....

He and I are in a strange, unwanted competition for the boys' affection.

117 From the kitchen, Muzzer sees that the light is on in the breezeway and automatically presses one of the illuminated red buttons on the kitchen wall, casting me into darkness. She will do so several times during the evening.

118 If it were a case of rewiring his sons, he could have handled it. What he can not handle is their diminishing light, a dimming he can in no way correct.

119 His office is his home. His spirit travels.

Above the television, a shelf displays miniature replicas of the three ships that sailed to the new world: the *Nina*, the *Pinta* and the *Santa Maria*. Each has a small light in its sail. At either end of the shelf sit copper ship lamps, one with a green light, the other blue: port and starboard.

On an L-shaped shelf in the corner behind the desk is a collection of miniature jet aircraft, each one raised upon its own short stand, as though in flight.

Boss has taken more than one vacation on his own, to Holland. The most recent was shortly after our arrival in New Jersey in September. On a low shelf behind his desk stand several large, three-ring binders, with the initials CVR embossed on their covers. The binders carefully lay out, day by day, the paper trail of each trip, with tickets, brochures, postcards and receipts, and photographs of places and friends.

120   He does not have many visitors to his office-apartment, but Uncle Lauw usually comes once a week, for an hour on Sunday mornings, after church.

The brothers spend most of Lauw's visit in the small utility room between the office and the front yard. Boss's smoking antechamber. Its walls have taken on a dull brown colour and look as though a fly might stick to them.

Lauw makes a brief appearance in the house before leaving, to visit the boys. He shows his face, as Eric puts it.

Loud and blustery, his humour forced, he exudes the desire to get out of the living room as quickly as possible. He seems embarrassed to be there.

121   Boss calls his daughter Mary Ann, or, with both letters distinctly enunciated, M. A.

While she was in high school and still living at home, she emerged in the morning from her basement room into the kitchen. The electrician was drinking coffee at the counter, waiting for the hoisting call, waiting for his daughter, and he would sing, as in the beauty pageant:

"Here she comes, Miss America...."

He struck her, once.

One July 4th weekend, on the day of the family picnic at Goffle Brook Park, Boss wanted to get the lawn cut. He made a wrong move with the mower and accidentally severed the big toe of his right foot. He hobbled over to the front door and banged on it, but when Mary Ann went to answer she saw blood on the window, and ran away.

That's not when he hit her. He hit her later, reflexively, when she accidentally stepped on his missing big toe while the foot was still in bandages.

122 Early Saturday afternoons Boss visits the Dutch store in town and selects supplies for an Indonesian feast of nasi goreng, or bahmi, dishes which he learned to create while with the Dutch merchant marine in Indonesia. He spends a good part of the afternoon preparing the meat-rich meal, which includes as appetizer a kind of flat, shrimp chip, which expands to enormous size in a pot of hot oil. He is expansive, and clearly enjoys doing this. He is using the presence of Mary Ann and me in the house to do something he would otherwise not have the opportunity or excuse to do. Mumphy cannot shed her air of mild disapproval, though she tries not to let it show. Boss simply ignores her, his one foot propped on the kitchen chair as he stirs the food in the electric frypan.

He also makes a mean bean soup.

The boys gamely try their father's cooking. They don't want to disappoint him. Their mother has prepared them a milder, backup meal, just in case.

123 Grandma stands in the hall with her coat on, a jar of leftover rice pudding nestled in her arm, and says out loud, "Okay, I'm ready to go. Who's driving me home?"

Two or three times a week Grandma comes for dinner. After dinner she reads the Paterson Evening News, does a crossword puzzle and plays a game of Scrabble with Paul. She and Grandpa played Scrabble almost every evening and kept numerous booklets and sheets of paper with their scores on them in the box. The boys tallied up their win/loss percentage and the total scores of all their years of playing. The couple were within two or three games of each other, with very few points separating them.

She is not a competitive player. She does not look for the big word score, but plays any letters on her rack that will make a word that fits the first place she sees open on the board. When it's not her turn she hums tunes, hymns mostly, or sings nonsense syllables, *do dah do do*, and taps her fingers on the arm of the chair or the tabletop. She's in her own world, and entirely content to be there.

Nine o'clock. Grandma is ready to go home.

"Who won the Scrabble game?" her driver asks.

"Oh, I don't remember any more."

"Your memory isn't what it used to be."

"No, when you get old you can't keep things in your mind so easily."

The drive home is along streets she has travelled almost all of her life. She points out where her cousins live. Where Aunt Alice lives. Asks if the driver wants to join the Army as the car passes the recruiting office. After the turn up Hill Street, she does *not* say "Did you ever see so many birdhouses?" at the house on the corner, where an array of homemade birdhouses is displayed. But only because it is night. And only because it is night, she says nothing about the brilliant reds and yellows of the houses. Lack of daylight, however, does not prevent her from commenting on the colour of one of the houses farther up the street.

"I would never paint my house that colour, would you?"

Just before the turn into her own driveway she nods to the low, red house across the street, and says, "You know Mrs. Mohawk, across the street? Her brother-in-law Frank took out the garbage one night, and he must have had a stroke while he was carrying it out. They found him the next morning, frozen dead solid."

Her widowed sister lives next door. Aunt Sue will wait until the shade in Clara's bedroom is drawn before going to bed herself. If the same shade is not up again by ten in the morning, she will go to see if anything is wrong.

She has found the key in her purse and is gripping it in her hand as she walks. The headlights of the car shine the length of the driveway, giving Grandma the light she needs to see her way, to find the keyhole in the back door. She is a small, bent, frail woman, moving slowly and deliberately along the side of a house that looks huge beside her, watching the ground, holding the handrail as she climbs the steps up to the enclosed porch. These are the same steps that Mary Ann climbed on Saturdays as a child to spend a morning learning to sew and knit, to have a lunch prepared especially for her, and to enjoy undivided adult attention.

Grandma turns the key in the lock and enters. The car doesn't back out until the light inside the porch brightens the windows.

124 Upstairs in Grandma's house there is one finished room, where Fran's brother slept. The rest of the space is open, attic-like, with exposed rafters and roof sheathing, the shingle nails poking through, and the smell of wood dried to baking from the summertime heat on the roof. It has served as play area for children and grandchildren.

Inside the room, in a closet, stands a four-drawer dresser. Painted battleship grey, with cherry-red drawer fronts and attached mirror, it inspired fear and exerted an irresistible pull on Mary Ann. Inside the top drawer lay a curled fox fur, all head and black nose and glass eyes, and softness.

125 FRIDAY NOV. 25

1. John got me out of stall at 9:27
2. E. meandered into L.room at 10:31
3. Mrs.VanDenBerg came at 12:46 + left at 4:02 4. We completed 30 out of 33 in the passing. 5. We did play by play of the first half of the Knicks-Celtics game. The Celtics were leading 79-50 at half time. 6. Neil went to the hospital. The ambulance left the house at 10:15. 7. Mumphy layed down from 2:37 to 3:55.

126 Neil returning to the hospital meant that the house had a satellite location. Mumphy travelled back and forth between the two. Now she had two jobs.

127 A week after the new routine began, Eric began having trouble breathing after his treatment. He also couldn't spit up the phlegm the inhalator usually freed. We waited until later in the evening, when Mumphy came home from the hospital, then called the police, who came to the house with a tank of oxygen. Eric used up the tank, and the police retrieved another from their car. By then the ambulance corps had arrived with additional tanks.

As many as ten people were standing in the bedroom while Eric, sitting up in bed, tried his best with the oxygen. Whenever the call goes out, a full contingent of police and ambulance corps and firefighters responds. A collective memory is at work. Everyone understands what has been going on in this family, in this house, for the past twenty years. No one can do anything about it. What they can do is come when there is need. And they do, in numbers, at a moment's notice.

Not one of the ten standing in the room could change places with him, could give him their body, or breathe for him. He was completely alone, and completely dependent on the people who stood helpless around him.

Eric naturally felt embarrassed about all the attention. He's a radio, rather than a television personality, after all. But he remained ever the verbal opportunist. While trying to cough up the phlegm, with the oxygen mask in the hand of the corps member standing beside him, he threw a sly look up at the attendant and, for the benefit of the crowd, said:

"I think I'll have another round."

Finally, at 11:30, he was taken to the hospital.

Paul, sitting up in his own bed, had remained uncharacteristically quiet the whole time.

Mary Ann reported later that before we left for the hospital, Eric said to his brother, "I know you're praying for me, Bull, and it makes me feel better."

128 Eric stayed in hospital for two days. Three days before Christmas he was admitted again, for the same reasons, but returned home on Christmas Eve.

Neil, though, remained in hospital through Christmas and into the New Year. It eventually became his third, six-week stint. Not until the end of December was he able to breathe without the respirator.

With two of the boys in hospital, Mumphy spent the entire day there, doing what the nurses would normally not have time for, which included keeping them comfortably positioned in bed, and helping Neil eat. Various volunteers also went to the hospital.

129 It was an odd Christmas anyway. We opened gifts early.

Boss received an omelet pan, an apron and spices, and a chocolate letter B. Mumphy received cookies, an invitation to lunch, a blouse.

Eric received a New York Knicks hat, a pad of paper with a pig on the cover, and a wooden microphone I'd carved for him; Paul a Chicago Bulls hat, more paper for his diary notebook, and a bull head that I'd also carved.

Grandma received a flannel nightie, fruit and a subscription to TV Guide.

Mary Ann received a mug and a hand mixer; I, a decent pair of slacks, a rake for my unruly hair and Band-Aids.

The volunteer firemen, as they did every Christmas, came with gifts for the boys. A stopwatch for Eric, a Scrabble game for Paul, and they visited Neil in the hospital with blank tapes.

Mary Ann and I flew home. We experienced a family Christmas like those we had enjoyed over the previous three winters of living in Ontario, though we were no longer so at ease in the old dispensation.

130   When guests had come for our wedding, they were given driving directions through the winding web of roads that is northern New Jersey. One friend in particular savoured the unusual sounds of the place names: HoHoKus, Mahwah, Weehawken, Tappan Zee. One day early in the new year, I was remembering that as Mumphy, Mary Ann, Paul, Eric and I made our way to an orthopaedic supply store in Hackensack.

We were in Hackensack following the suggestion that a custom brace, something like a rigid vest, might help support the boys' upper body weight. As their muscles became more lax and unable to support that weight, their organs were being crushed in the slump of their torsos while they sat in their wheelchairs or in bed, which aggravated their problems in sitting comfortably and breathing.

The two attendants mixed up the plaster and gauze. We hoisted Paul up into a sitting position on a doctor's office-style, padded table. I climbed onto the table behind Paul, wrapped an arm under each of his arms, and raised him, holding him as stretched upward as possible, as the attendants began winding and wrapping the sodden gauze around his torso. He had to be held in that stretched position for as long as it took for the plaster to set. Then the cast was sawn off and they had the mould that would produce a brace.

Then came Eric, a heavier lift.

The process was physically taxing for all, and everyone harboured secret doubts as to whether a brace would help. The entire effort seemed an exercise in futility, a grasping after straws.

Our orthopaedic adventure lasted from 9:30 in the morning to 5:30 in the afternoon. A Thursday.

131 Watching me limp along, someone asked, "Fighting the angel again?"

The pain was in my hip and down my leg to the knee. I took stairs one at a time, lifted my leg into and out of the car. For a few nights I could lay in only one position in bed, on my back, and would wake whenever my body wanted to roll over. The night was a big, empty bus that stopped at each stop along its route, opened its doors and let its light spill onto the sidewalk, closed its doors with a sigh and moved on, still empty. I experienced sleep as a long, frequently interrupted journey, alone.

But how could I have missed it? How could it not have occurred to me, when I was waking up during the night because I wanted to turn over in my sleep, but couldn't turn over because of the discomfort, the pain, and had to try to go back to sleep in the same position, how could it not have come to mind over those three or four nights that what I was experiencing my three brothers had experienced every night, thirty years ago?

132 Paul wanted to do his part for his own care and maintenance. The retention of fluids was an issue for all three of the boys. Starting in December, he had been recording in his diary his daily ounces of intake and output, together with the number of times he'd used the urinal.

"Friday: input 82 ounces, output 63 ounces."

After Neil came home from the hospital, Paul decided that his diary should have no more entries documenting his use of the urinal.

The two events are not obviously related.

133 Paul has decided that he should watch less television.

Normally, the two boys are prepared for bed shortly after dinner, and hoisted onto their mattresses before the evening games begin. Basketball, baseball, football. They know the teams well enough to be able to turn off the television sound and provide their own coverage. Ike "Behind-the-Mike" White provides the play-by-play. Willie puts his two cents into a more general commentary on the players, the quality of the game, a comparison of teams and seasons.

If Willie has decided on a career change, Ike will need to make accommodations. He'd never look for another sidekick: Willie is irreplaceable.

The brothers' problem came down to sight and sound. They put their heads together for a solution. Boss produced a sheet of cardboard and was instructed to wedge it between the mattress and the footboard of Paul's bed, solving problem number one by blocking Paul's view of the television. Earphones plugged into the television jack, its wire stretching to the bed, solved problem number two.

Eric listens to the games, compiling and sorting the growing heap of numbers, in silence. Ike has taken an early retirement from behind the microphone in aid of his brother's quest.

Paul reads the Bible and devotional literature; thinks and prays. He does not say, but chances are he is thinking and praying about others: the volunteers, helpers, nurses and their families who come to the house. Their extended families. He has developed an insatiable appetite and concern for the lives of everyone he meets.

It is very quiet in Paul and Eric's room in the evening, now.

The brothers are separating.

134 In the photograph, Eric sits on a chair that is fixed to a piece of plywood on wheels. He is leaning over the bathroom sink. Behind him, a homemaker, Mrs. Tchinnis, holds a waiting washcloth.

A practical intimacy. An everyday occurrence. Doors do not need to be closed, in fact they ought not to be closed in case help is needed. He might just as easily be sitting on the toilet. There is, in fact, an earlier photo of Neil sitting slung in the strap of the mechanical hoist, hanging in the air over the toilet.

The look on Eric's face is comic, pseudo-shock; mugging for the camera.

Mrs. Tchinnis has a good sense of humour, plays along.

She and her husband, who are both in their early sixties,
approaching retirement, go out dancing most weekends.
We learned this about her almost by accident. We want to
know more, but she is reluctant to talk about it, and refuses
to be coaxed.

135 Sometimes the smell that comes from a bathroom will
bring everything back.

The smell that does this is not the direct, powerful odour
but rather the smell that lingers after cleaning-up. It's the
scent that has slipped past, escaped cleansing, though
often it is mixed together with that of ammonia or bleach.
The one scent will evoke the other will evoke the memory of
the house and its daily functioning. This is not the smell of
the nursing home; not the urine smell of people who have
lost some bladder control. It is also not a hospital smell.
In part, it is the smell of three young men, of humanity,
vying against a necessary quest for cleanliness, a quest that
does not realize that it may also, unknowingly, be trying
to obliterate all traces of what the three young men cannot
control, which is to say the direction that their bodies are
travelling.

A quest that is trying with relentless vigour to exert
control in the one area where it can, in the cleanliness
of material objects, at least partly because it has so little
control over the things that are so much more important.

That is to say, there is nothing she can do about the
physical destiny of her three sons.

136 During the initial examination, the chiropractor remarked that damage to my back was causing a problem with the sciatic nerve that ran down my leg. The damage had likely occurred at least fifteen years earlier.

A ladder had slipped out from underneath me about that long ago, and I'd landed on it, full force, and fractured two elbows. Could that have done it?

Possibly, the chiropractor said.

I'd had to stand, not kneel, behind Paul, and then Eric, and lean over and forward and lift them, in order to allow the two attendants at the orthopaedic clinic room to wind the gauze around their torsos. And then hold them upright for ten, fifteen minutes, until the plaster set. That was twenty-five years ago. How about twenty-five years ago? I asked. Could the damage have been done then?

Possibly, the chiropractor said.

I would like the damage to have been done then.

137 Paul experiences breathing problems. The ambulance is called.

Calling the ambulance has become such a common occurrence that we enjoy a friendship with the attendants as you would with any person who regularly comes to the door as part of their work. A mail carrier, for instance.

And Paul is only too happy to be the one now admitted into the hospital. He is only too pleased to be assigned to the mission field of a general ward.

138 Paul is obviously in his element later that evening, when Mary Ann and I visit.

Sitting up in bed, inquiring after the attending nurse's elderly father, learning the stories of the other patients in the room from her. He'd caught up earlier with the afternoon nurse, whom he remembered from his first stay in the hospital, almost a year ago, finding out how things had worked out with a teenage son who played football and had been going through a difficult time.

We leave when visiting hours end.

See you tomorrow, Bully.

The Bull sends his low, bull bellow out of the room with us. Following us down the hallway till we are out of earshot, we hear *So looong Mary Ann, So looong Johnnny.*

139 It came as a complete surprise.

The phone rang at two o'clock a.m. Mary Ann groped to pick up, heard, "Valley Hospital", and hung up, thinking someone had dialled a wrong number. It rang again, and by this time she'd woken up enough to know that the voice was simply identifying itself.

Paul had died. Respiratory failure. January 17, 1978.

Twenty-one years old. Not bad for a bull.

140 "It's better this way."

"He's in a better place."

The effect of the condolences is cumulative. Have the good people of this community been waiting for this eventuality, so that they can finally say aloud what has always been thought, that this one life was not, in the end, preferable to its death?

141 Everyone thought Neil would be first. It seemed obvious that it would be Neil. He's the eldest, had been in the hospital so often, was so often critically ill. Even Neil thought it would be himself.

He's ready.

He does not want his brothers to suffer what he has had to suffer.

The reception after the funeral was held at the house. Neil lay in his bed down the hallway. People stopped by his room to share the sorrow, and to visit.

"I'm happy for Paul," he said.

142 Neil didn't attend the service, of course, but neither did Eric. The minister, a man Neil's age, fresh out of seminary, for whom Paul's had been his first funeral, described the service to Eric.

When the minister got to the part about praying, Eric interjected,

"Did you put in a plug for me?"

143 The emptiness was profound. None of us imagined what not returning from the hospital would mean.

Paul's living room chair was taken off its rolling dolly for the reception, and its terry-towel cover removed. It looked like any other piece of furniture. How very odd for Paul's chair to be serving a formal role, as though it had not had a specific, daily use, up until now. The TV tray was folded away, too. Neither were returned to their positions in the days following. Neil's table had remained in place long after he'd become bedridden, though now it too had been put away. The living room looked half normal. Which only intensified the feeling of absence, even when people came to visit, or especially then, since Paul had been the conversationalist.

The whole house was much quieter without its family chatterer. He who could be so annoying, left a big hole. The thoughtful one, who asked to be pushed into his brother's room at the close of each day, so he could spend time with his isolated, elder kinsman. Mr. Conscientious. He had recently been dictating thank-you letters to former nurses, homemakers and volunteers.

144 Two members are now missing from the fraternal living room triumvirate, one down the hallway, one for all time. Only the quiet one remains at his station.

For Eric, it is like having a limb removed. Paul is his true alter ego, his other half. No pig or owl comes near his brother.

Eric is valiant, keeps up the show. The games continue; home and professional statistics are maintained.

He begins to consider his biography.

145 Life Behind The Mike
The Living Legend Of Ike White
by Isaac "Ike" White

CHAPTER 1: A BIT OF HISTORY

Isaac "Ike" White was born in the Baconville Memorial Hospital, in Buffalo, New York. When Ike was still a young piglet, he and his parents moved to Albany. Abraham White and his spouse Bertha were originally from Babbs and McWillie, Oklahoma, respectively. They met at the 1946 annual Church Picnic. Abraham was the judge of the bake-off, and he gave Bertha a blue ribbon for her cornpone, which he subsequently ate (Ike gets his appetite from his father). Though at the time a portly pig, Abe slimmed down considerably after meeting Bertha. They were married in 1948, after a two year courtship.

Abraham White was a Baptist preacher, and after their marriage he heard about a church in Buffalo that needed a preacher. So Bertha packed the bags and Abe started the car, and they left behind their home in Oklahoma. Bertha was getting plump at about this time, and they were expecting a piglet in the family. Isaac White was born on Aug. 25, 1950, at the stroke of midnight.

But Ike was a premature piglet. He weighed only 3lbs. 9oz., and had to be kept in an incubator for 24 days. Abe & Bertha came to the hospital every day. They spent a lot of their time in the waiting room, praying and wondering what would happen.

Ike passed the critical stage and soon started looking pink and healthy. They had hardly taken him home, however, when it turned out that Abe and Bertha would have to go live in Albany. Abe had accepted a call to one of the churches and so the Whites moved to the city of Ike's childhood years.

146 Eric dictated from behind his card table each afternoon.

Ike White wasn't interested in the glory. He felt the biography needed to be told. He owed it to his public.

His models came from the world of sport biography. His scribe sat on the couch with pad and pencil. His ghost writer. His hired gun. His "as told to" person. Eric had any one of a number of ways to describe what they were doing.

"I'm going to launch your career, Johnny."

147 I took this job long ago. What's kept me?

Johnny's been slacking off.

Johnny hasn't been able to do it, until now.

There is nothing here that comes near to describing their experience.

148 CHAPTER 2: IKE'S HIGH SCHOOL DAYS

Ike wasn't much of an athlete. He liked sports, but he knew he wouldn't be very good at them, so he figured out other ways to get involved. One thing he did was turn off the sound on the TV and do a play-by-play description of the game. He was also an umpire at Little League games.

Ike tried out for the football team in his freshman year. He made the team because without him they wouldn't have enough players. In practice they used him to hold the tackling dummy, so he became the key to their tackling success. He liked to think he was good, but as he later said, "Deep down I knew better."

His sophomore year, more kids turned out for the team, so Ike only got a chance to play on garbage time, when his team was winning by a mile or losing by two, and it didn't matter anymore. He spent so much time on the bench he got splinters.

The highlight of Ike's football career came in the last game of the season. Ike's team was leading 53 to 6, 2:45 left in the 4th quarter. When the coach called him into the game he felt stiff as a board and his feet had fallen asleep.

"Them" had the ball at their own 5 yard line. The quarterback faded back to pass. He was under a hard rush, but Ike wasn't the one who was rushing. The quarterback tried to throw a screen pass to his halfback. The ball hit Ike squarely on the helmet and bounced into his arms. He sprinted two yards and fell over the goal line. "At that point the game was ours. Actually of course they couldn't touch us anyway, but it meant a lot to me."

That was Ike's last time in uniform. "The game I'll never forget," he says.

149   The account goes on to describe Ike's career as a high-school ten-pin bowler.

He picked up the sport as a junior, and by his senior year

became something of a champion. His parents gave him a bowling ball for his birthday.

Abe and Bertha were concerned that bowling would interfere with their son's studies, but even with all the practising and active competition, Ike kept up his grades. He became an honour's student and graduated with flying colours.

The biography ends not long after his high school graduation. Later in life, Ike founded the Owl Orphanage, a charitable institution dedicated to the raising of healthy owls.

150 We returned to Hackensack twice in the following weeks to have Eric fitted for his new brace. The braces hadn't been ready before Paul died.

He was in the hospital again for a week, so first we had to wait for him to come home.

After the final fitting, a small accident while pushing Eric into the van to go home injured his shoulder. At first it seemed as though the shoulder might be dislocated. It turned out to be only bruised, but the pain, which was slow to go away, kept him from trying the brace for a few days.

Eric was determined to make use of the new aid. It came as two moulded halves, plastic shells, with soft foam interiors, and Velcro on the sides to strap them together. He began a daily regimen of having the brace put on in the morning, before he went into the living room.

He wanted to build up his stamina by staying in it for a bit longer each day.

His goal was to get to the point where he would be able to sit through an entire New York Mets home game.

151	The same procedure was used to get him into the brace as had been used to have the mould made. He was lifted from under his shoulders and held up as the brace was wrapped around his torso. It kept him more or less squeezed upright, like a girdle.

He looked unnatural and uncomfortable. He had lost weight already, and seemed to have lost more since the original fitting, so the brace didn't fit as well as it might have. He seemed almost suspended by his underarms, hanging from the top rim of the brace.

After a few minutes, he began to sweat, shedding more pounds before our eyes.

Boss turned away. He couldn't look. He had been finding it harder lately to bear seeing what was happening to his youngest son. The dwindling away. This made things worse. He spent even less time in the house.

152	The strain of being in the brace proved too much. Eric had to give it up. The problems with his breathing and lying in bed and getting seated comfortably persisted. His heart periodically launched into bouts of furious beating. Having a body was becoming, for the first time, a true burden. He was enjoying fewer and fewer stretches of time in which he could recover and be himself.

At the beginning of March he was admitted to hospital again.

Mary Ann and I spent much of the first day with him. For the first time Mary Ann was afraid. At home, she didn't want to answer the phone.

On the afternoon of the second day, Mumphy called

home from the hospital. Eric had died. Respiratory failure. March 7; seven weeks after Paul.

He was nineteen years old.

153   Would it be correct to say that you made them that way, that is to say, diseased? I have no problem saying that you made them. Do we say, then, that you made them as they were, that there is a divine image that they, their bodies, made manifest?

There was nothing lovely in their disease. Read: you make all things lovely.

Yet a loveliness of spirit and of flesh was upon them.

There was nothing desirable in what their disease did to their lives.

Yet their lives attracted.

154   It is not better this way. It is not better to not have Eric or Paul around. It is worse. It stinks.

No one said these words to those who came to comfort, either in the funeral home or at the reception afterward. The words should have been shouted.

And no matter what anyone may think, a household that revolves around the care and comfort of three young men in wheelchairs, in bed, is not a horror. Young men who rarely complained about their condition, their lot. Who transcended their condition.

People mistook the relief the caretakers might feel in being freer, with happiness.

155 And then there was one. Neil in his room, in the emptied
house.

But Neil had died already. More than once. He had
also come back, more than once. The elder, the one most
hospitalized, had outlived his two younger siblings. With
his brothers gone, his work was done.

He, and we, entered the long season of his waiting to be
taken up, to ascend.

156 I got a job.

Each morning, as Boss leaned over the kitchen counter
nursing his mug of coffee, he looked across the fenceless
backyards of the houses across the street. One of those
yards belonged to a carpenter. The carpenter's garage and
truck were a scene of activity at that time of the day, as he
assembled his tools and supplies.

I had too much time on my hands now, without the two
boys to spend it with, and soon found myself wearing a pair
of overalls, and swinging a hammer.

My career was launched. If only Eric could see me now.

157 Neil is closer in age to Mary Ann than to his two younger
brothers. He was born, as she, in the first flush of marriage
and children. His birth made the apartment in Prospect
Park too small. It was he and Mary Ann who played by the
piles of sand and in the gravel driveway of the new house
being built across from the grandparent's home.

It is he who prompted the family to veer off the turnpike.

You're driving along in your Vista Cruiser when one
of the kids says, I have to pee, so you pull over to stop,

and from then on suddenly it's no more highway but just winding roads no one else is travelling, up and down and over and around, forever until it ends.

Neil is not unaware of his responsibility. The first; the first of three: the one the other two would observe and learn from. Learn what to expect. They could see their immediate physical future in him.

He does not feel blameworthy – although perhaps he does, a little. He was given the role by virtue of birth. He had no hand in that.

He has carried the weight and banner of the first-born male, just as though his blood were royal.

158 The bedroom was small, eight-by-eight feet. It had a hospital bed, a bedside table, a dresser and a record player in it, as well as a wall-mounted television. The television was in the corner beside the window that overlooked the backyard, a backyard so shallow the view actually took in the backyards of the houses on the next street. If the late-May trees were not so lush, he might have been able to see Goffle Brook winding and turning a bend.

Someone loved the brook so much, they hand-built a wooden bridge over it. Someone else loved the brook so much, they destroyed the bridge.

Posters of sports figures, male and female, were tacked to Neil's walls. A female presence existed here that had not found a place in his younger brothers' lives. Poster-size reproductions of natural scenes alternated on the wall with the athletes. The mountains and fields included a phrase or sentence from scripture, imposed over a patch of open sky or on the pale waters of a lake.

An eight-by-ten photo of the figure-skater Dorothy Hamill, darling of the '76 Winter Olympics, stood in a frame on a shelf in the corner. Beside her, a smaller photo of a local hero, Andy the plumber, posing beside the basement furnace. Snapped when the water boiler that heated the house had broken down.

There were many photos of people taken standing beside their cars. These were shot at Neil's request, when the people came to visit, or left. He wished to place the person beside their symbol of mobility.

A collection of beer cans lined a shelf above the window. The cans were unopened, like his father's office collection of single-ounce liquor bottles.

159 There wasn't a lot of extra space in the room to move about, other than around the end of the bed. The visitor unfolded a metal chair, placed it beside the bed, and blocked the doorway. This assured a minimum amount of privacy. Some people read the Bible aloud for him, or read devotional literature, or played a game, especially Scrabble.

Neil's Scrabble board held each letter in place inside a plastic pocket, which made it possible to prop up the game at a fairly sharp angle on the bed table, and swing it into his line of vision.

His method of play was the opposite of Grandma's, although the two played together companionably and often. Humming tunelessly, she took less than a minute to play the first four-letter word she could organize from the letters on her rack, caring neither for placement nor point total.

Neil might take thirty minutes to play two letters in a

strategic location that gained him forty points, and jammed
the board for his opponent.

160 Neil had friends in a way that Paul and Eric did not, partly
because the two younger brothers had each other, partly
because by going to school longer he had spent more time
in the wider world. Male and female came. They'd close the
door and play records.

His record collection proved that he and I were of the
same generation and shared some of the same tastes.
"Worst of Jefferson Airplane," "Live at Leeds" by the Who;
many Youngbloods LP's. A pile of Bill Cosby's comedy
records, such as "Why Is There Air?", "To my brother
Russell, whom I slept with." I listen to these and wonder
why we didn't get to know each other better. I spent a lot of
time with the boys, less with him.

Neil spent more time in medical emergency, or being
attended to. That's the reason, Mary Ann assures me.

In order for him to breathe more easily, the cork was
usually removed from the trach in his throat. Talking was
a strain for him. He could manage no more than a whisper.
That's another reason, she says.

He was also more reflective, and might have told me what
it was really like.

I feared finding out what it was really like. That's the real
reason, I tell myself. There's a little Uncle Lauw in us all.

161 His was a physical presence in the way that his two brothers
were not. The presence of his disease, stretched out on the

bed, hips disjointed, legs akimbo, head and torso tilted
upward. A horizontal ballet. He'd been dancing this way for
a long time.

He lay there in the flesh, his flesh. His broken glory.
The body as landscape.

162   SCRABBLING FOR REPOSE

Beyond the bedroom wall, through the window,
hurried birds are pecking freely from the feeder.
Sparrow, grackle, wren, and a stubborn squirrel
who won't scare will winter under the eaves.
We keep it filled to keep them trained to keep
you entertained, I guess.

                              What is it
this or that side of the pane
most captivates your eye? the yard out back?
great with late summer
                              Flora Dea
her last fling
                    or the perfect landscape pictured
here
           where to the left another photo
shows a brook and underneath is printed
The hart panteth.
                         Do you stop and drink
Cornelius, and then, revived, focus
for a time on TV? or do you count
tomatoes, next door?
                              They ripened last
month, hanging red moons in hundreds

keeping the missus busy, bent over
filling baskets, her fingers calm and fast
into the plant, her buttocks round and swaying
swaying round the garden ground.

                          Do you take
by the way
          any interest in women? Is it her
physique
        invited Nadia Comanech
                   up
onto the wall? She contemplates the mat.
Steady and precise, and with a young body
she will wind between the branches of
the parallel bars, weave a routine from
pole to pole and land like a bird in
perfect perch
           scoring ten.
                   Beside her
Mercury Morris concentrates on hanging
there, reaching out his fingertips
to meet mid-air a pass that comes from somewhere
off the poster.
            Remember that game? He jumped
for nothing, landed out of bounds, no yards
third down, they decided to kick, and one
of the sixty thousand gathered there
                        caught the thing
and Sunday evening brought a football home.

      One time at the stadium, hoping to watch
the Mets win once, the pitcher tossed a ball
from the bullpen that landed on your lap.

He signed it first, and there it sits, name-
forward on the shelf.
                      Did he even play that game?
or was he, like you, consigned to sit out
all nine innings?
                   Where does your contract stipulate
how much you may or not participate?

The board game stands propped
                         perpetual
on the bed table. Seven letters
each, we drop words
               without sentence.
They lie in our silence like cyphered conversation
like clues to character and chance, like trachs
through which you cannot talk, meals
through a straw, like staring out the window
round the room, like victory
                  like victory
for you
        I've yet to win a single match
against this monumental calculating patience.

        Say it, Neil.
                  What dire sentence left
the tongue of God the day you were conceived?
Bedridden
           born to the interrogative
you leave us stand, begging.
We scrabble for repose
               while you
       wordlessly pursue.

163 The human body as landscape. Is that where this is heading? Neil as one of the shapes among which we move. The three brothers as exemplars of Nature flawed; the earth, hurting.

Neil became an example of another direction that a human being, a body, can take. One that surprisingly few do.

How is that so many are born whole and sound? How can it be that so few are born misshapen or with parts missing, or with parts in the wrong place? Why are there not more who are horribly disfigured? Or are millions born this way, but hidden away?

His body a temple on a hill. The temple of his twenty-four years. The hill of coiled metal springs, and foam padding.

Let the world come, see. Leave your canes by the door.

164 We are whole, single beings. No separation exists between body and soul. Brook no dualism. Thus had I been taught.

Neil looked forward to leaving his body behind. And told you so. Told us, too. His body was killing him, while he wanted to live. The part of him that wanted to live was therefore, for him, the not-body. The soul. Spirit.

He wanted out. He wanted free.

165 The body makes theologians of us all.

166 Boss went to a car dealership on Route 17 one Saturday morning. I watched amazed as he paid cash for a brand new Oldsmobile Delta 88. All those electrical house calls: cash jobs. He kept a locked box in his office.

We took the obligatory photograph of him standing beside it in the driveway.

The following weekend he drove the car, with its air conditioning, power brakes, power steering, power windows (non-standard features for the time), on its first highway run, north to Connecticut, to show off and visit his sister Co and her family. Many of her ten children were already married and had children. He was a great-uncle several times over.

167 Early on, Boss told a close friend that his world came to an end when he first received the news of his three sons' condition. His initial thought was to put them all in the car and drive into the river.

He said this only once.

168 Mary Ann and I walked to church on Sunday mornings. A tree-lined five or six blocks. We'd done so most of the fall and winter. Now it was warmer again. No matter how often we invited him to, Boss never accompanied us, preferring the car.

As we walked, cars slowed beside us on the road, and windows rolled down, and the Sunday heads inside offered us a ride. The scene repeated itself until we were within singing distance of the parking lot. In New Jersey no one walked by choice. If you were seen on foot, it meant that your car must have broken down. You'd welcome a lift.

Mumphy stayed home and listened to the service over the speakerphone, keeping Neil company.

We strolled home after the service to find her sitting at the kitchen table.

She sat slumped in the chair, her back to us as we walked in, and hardly turned or looked up to say that Neil had died during church. Kidney failure.

It was June 7. He was twenty-four.

169 Nothing looked different in his room. He was hardly less mobile than he had been. His breathing had stilled. His breathing: that barely discernible rising of his chest.

Impossibly, he lay there yet. The ceiling was in place. The room had not opened to the sky; the rafters were not charred and smoking. The prophet's flaming chariot had not come down to carry Neil to heaven.

We should have been standing beside an empty bed, squinting after him, into the clouds.

Don't you think that would have been the right thing?

170 We didn't call Boss in Connecticut. It seemed unnecessary. Neil's death was not unexpected. No one wanted to spoil Boss's brief vacation, and he'd be home later in the evening anyway.

Now it seems unfair. Corey talks and drinks coffee with his sister, his nieces and nephews, their children. He's the uncle, the great uncle, any kid would love to have. Then he drives his new car for three hours, flowing down the turnpike through the Hudson River valley as smoothly as the river itself.

The post-light by the driveway is shining for him.

We hear the slam and clatter of the jalousies in the breezeway door, and then the door into the kitchen opening.

171 Was death reaching back from where it normally takes its stand, at the end of life, back to birth? Reaching back from the point where we walk into its arms, naturally, slowed to a stop by old age? Farther back than the tragic car accident in mid-life, or the accidental drowning as a teenager, the fever that turns suddenly fatal for the young child? Back farther than the stillborn baby? Was death reaching into the womb itself, the cup of life, and to the very moment of conception?

What did it want, death? Was it trying to snatch these three from the hand of the giver of life? From the hand of life itself? To claim them as its own from the first moment of their existence?

How dextrous of death, how able. How we should congratulate it on getting there first.

Only it didn't get there first. First there was the attraction that brought the two human beings together, that sparked the fire by which the third was created. All death could do at that point was watch, and long, and wish.

And tamper with the tiny flame.

172 No one had spoken of it, of how sure their three deaths were. Death was denied the recognition it had placed right in front of everyone's face, in the very middle of everyone's life, in the boys' very bodies. A recognition it had gone to such extraordinary lengths to receive. They simply refused to acknowledge its presence or its power.

And they all died.

Death where is thy sting? In the sciatic nerve. In surviving.

173 "They're in a better place."

"They're probably playing a three-on-one on heaven's basketball court."

"Now you can build your own life again."

174 What is life? What is *a* life?

Mary Ann and I stayed in New Jersey with Boss and Mumphy through July. During that time, a couple from Holland came to visit, younger than Boss, but old friends of his, whom he regularly visited on his solo trips to his home country. Boss had known Frans for a long time. Frans had been babysat by Boss's sister. He had also served as a porter on a ship when he was young. When his ship docked in New Jersey, he came to visit. He'd known the boys almost since they were born.

Boss felt very much at home with both Frans and Gretha, joked around and showed an ease and enjoyment that his daily life otherwise did not elicit.

The six of us all fit into the new Delta 88, and together we travelled for a few days into Pennsylvania and the Pocono Mountains.

175 *The Ballad of Nine-toed Fathers.*

My father, meanwhile, was convalescing in a lounge chair on his backyard patio in Ontario.

Early in July, he wanted to get the lawn cut quickly before leaving for a holiday. He backed the mower over his foot and lost the big toe on his left foot.

Boss had lost the big toe on his right foot.

Mary Ann and I pondering the cryptic oddity of what we shared.

176 Boss and Mumphy began to build their life together. They travelled. They came to visit us for a few days in our second-floor flat, back in Canada. We gave them the hometown tour. Showed them where we worked. Sat at the kitchen table, ate and talked, played cards.

I had come to respect my father-in-law more and more. He either did not notice or refused to notice, or was content to wait until the day when Mumphy came around – if she came around. But he was loyal, did not give up.

And he did not cease to seize and relish the moment, especially those moments in the company of others.

177 It is possible to read Mumphy's lack of participation, her almost-indifference, as an aspect of her piety, an implicit form of judgment, or as the dulling of her spirit brought on by three deaths, part of the long process of getting-over-it.

Why is it so difficult not to judge her for it?

178 They made a trip to Holland, and stayed with Frans and Gretha, who owned an old home beside a dike, outside of Rotterdam. Boss quit forty years of smoking in the weeks

prior to the trip, because he did not want to tempt Gretha, who had recently quit.

He sat on their couch one morning with a cup of coffee while Gretha prepared breakfast. He didn't feel well. He didn't look well. Frans called the next-door neighbour, who was a nurse. The nurse immediately called the doctor, who was a friend. The doctor immediately called an ambulance.

Frans asked Fran, through the bathroom door, if she wished to come along to the hospital. Nothing to worry about, he told her. Still in the process of waking up and washing herself, she said that she would remain home.

Boss was talking to Frans as he, like his sons before him, was lifted into the ambulance. He would spend some time in the hospital, get thoroughly checked up, and be better. That seemed clear.

179   He'd had a heart attack on the couch in the living room.

In the hospital he had a second, more severe attack, and died. It was April 23, 1980. Two years after his sons. He was fifty-nine. The same age as his father.

180   Mumphy made the complicated arrangements to have Boss's body transported across the ocean, home for the funeral. Frans accompanied her. Boss's brothers and sisters flew from the west coast. We hadn't seen them for years.

It seemed all too familiar, standing in the funeral line, receiving condolences.

After the funeral the three of us returned to the house, alone.

181 Dying of old age was the privilege granted to Grandma, six months later – six weeks after she entered a nursing home.

With her mother's death, Mumphy no longer had any family living near. She took a secretarial course, but after graduating decided not to look for a job but do volunteer work instead. She'd discovered that she could live on the income from investments and the rent of Boss's office as a bachelor apartment.

She sent us weekly letters with the church bulletin folded inside it, newspaper clippings, and detailed menus from meals at friends' homes.

She came to visit two or three times a year, by bus, as our children were born and grew. They spent early mornings in her bedroom, sharing animal crackers and religious tracts. We broke down and bought our first television set, so that she wouldn't have to rely on updates of her favourite soap opera from a neighbour when she returned home. That same soap opera, after all these years.

In the evenings, the tiny mirror balanced on her lap, the familiar cough-drop tin of bobby pins lay within handy reach, as she put her hair up in pincurls.

Prior to each of these visits, Mary Ann and I would vow not to become impatient with Mumphy's habits and quirks. Within five minutes of her arrival, we were already becoming testy. The testiness deepened during the length of her stay.

Each time the bus doors wheezed shut behind her and she was on her way home to New Jersey, we regretted our inability to rise above the petty irritations.

182 As a grandma, Mumphy told one small joke. It came from a time before her marriage, when she was working in an office in Paterson and shopped downtown, went roller skating and shared lunch hours with a girlfriend.

It wasn't a joke, but word play, and totally out of character, or what we thought was her character. Following thanks before a meal, for the benefit of her two granddaughters, she would echo the closing Amen with, "Ah, men!"

183 Returning home during winter break from college, the year we married, Mary Ann wrote in a journal:

MARCH 20

Home again. It's great to be pampered a little. Coming home is finding a box of Valentine's candies on your bed from your mother who tells you why she got it. She says because it was on sale. Would have cost her $6.00 if she had bought it before February 14th.

"Well, it was marked down to $3.50 on the 27th, down to $2.50 on the 6th and just last Friday I saw it for $1.25. You were coming home and it does stay fresh in that cellophane – well, it was a real bargain."

Coming home is finding a real bargain on your bed and clean sheets underneath it.

184 While we were yet in college, Mary Ann and I decided that when the time came we would adopt children. The genetics of Duchenne muscular dystrophy ran against us. Males usually contracted the disease; females carried it. Mary herself was a carrier. If we had biological children, a boy stood a fifty/fifty chance of being born with it. A girl had the same odds of being a carrier.

No one would wish either of these situations on another human being. We were happy to be able to stop the disease in its generational tracks.

We sat in the specialist's office a few months before our marriage. The specialist told us we were too young to make a decision that would affect the rest of our lives, that we couldn't undo.

We talked to the family doctor. The doctor talked to the specialist, who then agreed to perform the procedure.

We were twenty-one years old. In terms of life expectancy for someone born with the disease, we were not the advanced age of Neil or the two boys, but as family we were old enough, and aging rapidly.

185 The day we spoke to the specialist was toward the end of Neil's first six-month stay in intensive care.

The doctor who spoke to the specialist on our behalf was about to, or perhaps had already cast the deciding vote on whether or not to pull the plugs on Neil's life-support machines. He had been the family's doctor since the boys were young.

Neil lived another four years.

186 A neighbour spotted Fran standing on the roof of the house.

Fran had put out a ladder, climbed up and was leaning forward over the edge of the roof, squatting in the dormer valley, cleaning it and the gutters of leaves.

This same neighbour remembers being surprised by and admiring Fran when the boys were still on their feet, and later on wheels. Admiring that Fran let the boys do pretty much whatever they wanted. She didn't restrain or protect them. And if one of them got into trouble or fell, there always seemed to be someone around to lift them up and hold them, swaying, as they caught their balance again and locked into position. Or to haul one of them out of hanging in the bushes.

The neighbour admired the young mother's fearlessness.

Fran moves from one spot on the roof edge, to the next. I can see her. She does the same in her yard. She does the same in our yard. Picking at the leaves, a stray twig here, a windblown piece of paper there.

She spent the better part of an afternoon pulling weeds in our yard, and inadvertently pulled out a three-foot high tree we'd nurtured from its planting by a squirrel.

"I wondered why that one was so hard to pull out," she said.

She has a curious, somewhat stiff gait. Herky-jerky, side-stepping, a form of waddling. As though her limbs were pulled by strings. As though whoever controls the strings is not adept. Where, in the shape of her body, are the shapes of the bodies of her sons?

187 The beauty of my mother.

188 A second entry from Mary Ann's journal:

MARCH 21

My mother is the kind of woman who when you give her a new set of dinner china for her anniversary first says thank-you and then wonders out loud whether or not her old set is still open stock and could have been supplanted instead. And even when you offer to pack the still good pieces away, she would rather pack in the creamer with one crack than throw it away with the other broken pieces – just in case. "Just in case you'll ever need some dishes. One crack isn't that noticeable. See it doesn't leak! Besides, what would you do with a sugar without a creamer?"

189 It never bothered us, neither personally nor as a couple, that we would have no biological children. Even for a minute.

Occasionally I've wondered if a minute would come, bringing with it regret, but none has. The grace given to Mary Ann to bear these things – and much grace has been given – I received a measure of. This is not self-commendation, but fact.

The fact and experience of her family has placed us together on the far side of regret.

For me, it would be as though to regret the love of my youth. The love that saved me.

190 Your mystery is contained in our individuality.
   Wonderfully and fearfully made.

And the making so personal. For some it is *very* personal, and so physical, it hurts.

191 The laborious and exacting science of placing the puck precisely where Neil's limited swing could strike to best advantage is matched only by the science of placing each of the three brothers in their wheelchairs in exactly the right position on the linoleum rink of the bedroom.

Move me a bit forward, Johnny, and straighten out my front wheels.

Move my left foot so it's out of the way. Back an inch.

Now turn my right back wheel so I'm at an angle.

That's too far, better back up. That's good. Now straighten my front wheels again.

I think that's it. Let's see.

He takes a practice shot to make sure the positioning is right. *Bully scores!*

Put the brakes on, Johnny.

Are you ready, tyrants?

Them's the breaks, Johnny.

So he's set for now, with minor adjustments as we play, and the other two go through the same routine. It is not difficult, but time-consuming and sometimes exasperating.

They are vitally concerned with their positions on the ice, with the overall balance in relation to each other, to their skills.

They are vital.

Thirty shots on goal each. Statistics compiled afterward by Eric.

192 On the kitchen table, between the toaster and the pencil mug, among the empty envelopes, Mary Ann found an advertising flyer for The Clothes Den (offering 10% off), on which Fran had pencilled the beginnings of a family biography:

"Their hearts were light, and we tried to live as normal a life as possible."

193 After the initial hesitation of a newcomer to the house, in the wake of repeated bruising from the three-iron, the goalie shows no mercy in the net, hurling verbal abuse and derogatory remarks at the three players.

Which they enjoy, and clearly intended to provoke from the start. A counterbalance to the abuse they are taking from their own bodies. The only roughhousing they can handle.

On his shins, the marks of their abandon.

As close as they can come to the physical abandon of the sport.

194 The question, first asked in high school, *What are you going to do?* meaning, *with your life,* and its deadly underlying riddle, *How are you planning to justify your existence on a day-to-day basis?* left me dumbfounded.

"Isn't it enough that I *am*?"

The boys proved it. The simple fact of your created being is sufficient for all time.

They proved it by being themselves and having no "future."

195 Paul and Eric each had a shorter version of the regulation hockey stick, with the famous *Victoriaville* stamped on its length. Neil's golf club was their ingenious solution to his difficulties in stickhandling.

They tried a wooden disc as a puck, but it proved dead on the floor.

They experimented with a street hockey ball, but it didn't stay in place for their slapshots, and rolled under beds and dressers all the time.

They tried the plastic cap of an aerosol can, from their mother's hairspray. It had the right weight for them to be able to fire a decent shot on goal, and enough bounce to deflect off the goalie and skip about on the floor in front of them without travelling too far (usually), which kept the game interesting.

And of the efficacious cap, a dozen filled their dresser drawer.

196 During a phone call with her daughter, almost fifteen years after she buried her eldest son, Fran said:

"I'm so depressed. I don't think that I ever really accepted the boys' deaths."

197 She called on the telephone from the hospital once when the paramedics were unable to get her blood pressure reading. They stood beside her as she talked.

The doctor told us to come to New Jersey.

Fran's brother and sister from Michigan came too, and helped to pull the necessary strings, to nudge the communal memory (it had been fifteen years since the boys' deaths) and have Fran admitted into the private health care facility where she had long ago worked as a practical nurse. There were no rooms available. A lounge was converted for her use.

The night nurse called to say we should come.

We sat on either side of her bed and waited as she breathed her last. Her shallow breathing simply ceasing.

198 We cleaned and rented out the house. When the time came to sell it, we returned to New Jersey to give the keys and the garage-door opener to the lawyer.

We sat together on the breezeway steps, going over all the good reasons why we had chosen not to live in New Jersey when we first married, or when her brothers had died, or two years later, when her mother found herself alone and without family.

All that afternoon, our ten-year-old daughter played by the brook that ran beside and behind the house, as her mother before her had, and her mother's mother. She came up to where we sat in the twilight.

"I can't get enough of this place," she said.

Some of Mary Ann's childhood friends had moved away simply because of the area's high cost of living. She and I moved to Toronto after we married, a young couple starting out on our own, and our lives had become interwoven with friends, with my family, and with the place itself.

There were no reasons good enough to absolve us. We chose.

Was it so that she, so that we, could leave behind, rather than be left behind?

199   New Jersey had seemed exotic from the start.

Lush with trees, roads winding up and around the many hills, beside brooks, through one small town after the other, densely populated but feeling rural all the same, built up piece by piece, over a long period of time: a populated paradise.

Everyone seemed to have constructed their own houses, or hired a carpenter to do so.

The community was at least two generations older than the one I grew up in, its levels of interrelatedness much more involved and complex, with extended family up to and beyond second cousin, once removed.

I liked everyone I met.

And New Jersey was home to the boys, their natural habitat.

200   Mary Ann enjoyed the orderly household she entered when she first visited Ontario.

Our family ate together, at a table, three meals a day. Coffee was served at ten-thirty in the morning, tea mid-afternoon, coffee again mid-evening, always with cookies or cake, always served with style and manners, though not overly formal.

My parents immigrated from Holland, and an awareness of Dutch culture existed in our language and food, and in the decor. We had little silver teaspoons, a thick rug on the coffee table, a few Delft pieces, and brass artifacts made from World War Two artillery shells.

My father and mother involved themselves in the wider community outside the home, in the church and school.

My father presided over their boards, over the board of the Dutch credit union. My mother taught adult night-school classes in macramé.

Ours was uncomplicated by more extended family. Mary Ann was welcomed into it wholly.

My home seemed *normal* to her, and therefore exotic.

201   The dresser that revealed a fox fur to a young girl is no longer painted battleship grey and cherry red. Its revealed grain evokes the trees on Hill Street, on the dead-end street that ran off a dead-end street, and the street-light pole at the corner, its isolated island of illumination on pavement and foliage.

The dresser drawers no longer stick or sag, their bottoms are not cracked or split. Using skills sharpened over the years, I fixed them.

And it is heartening that this restored piece of furniture should be with us in such an everyday fashion, its drawers sliding open, sliding shut.

As most of the material world of Mary Ann's childhood and youth has de-materialized.

202   He was installing a reception desk he'd made, filling nail holes with a wax crayon, Minwax #6, which made the nail holes stand out even more than they did unfilled, but which would eventually match the colour of the cherrywood, as the wood darkened with age. The receptionist was answering the phone at her makeshift station in another room, while one of the counsellors sat on the couch in the

reception area and asked if they, meaning the carpenter and his wife, had gotten away this summer.

Well, yes, he said, they'd gotten away, and explained that they had spent two weeks five hundred miles away, and had sat beside his wife's mother as she breathed her last breath. Literally.

"How's your wife taking it?" the counsellor asked.

The carpenter offered, awkwardly, that his wife had been "taking it" her whole life. He then provided the general outlines of the family narrative, the fact that her mother's leaving left her as the only surviving member of the family.

"What a tragedy," the counsellor said.

"Tragedy?"

203 Why did it never occur to me to ask why one family should be struck so?

Why should it? They were not my brothers after all.

They became my brothers the moment my arm reached around their sister's shoulder as we walked together and she told strange and wonderful accounts of their misadventures.

It would have been natural to ask. But so many people were asking why about so many different situations and circumstances, and were using the question as a way of blaming, of holding you responsible for what often seemed obviously the result of human action, or the free workings of nature.

But this disease was not the result of either of those, was it? I don't know. Perhaps it was both. Environmental pollution can have secret, mutating effects. The waters of

New Jersey are not innocent. As a young girl Fran swam in the pond created by the mill dam behind the house where she later lived as a mother of four. Could that have had something to do with it?

There is no answer to the question of where the disease came from or why one family was struck so.

Ask a different question.

Ask after the boys' liveliness, their imperishable life.

204 *It ain't why why why…it just is.*

The words lose something in the translation from being sung to being strung out in a line of type.

There is pain and ecstasy in the singing.

205 Waiting for the electrician's daughter.

Standing under the dormitory window in the snow waiting for her window to go dark and for her tall form to appear in a flood of light through the fire-escape door. So we may walk together. Walk and talk under the stars whirling on their silent and sleepless axis.

Waiting to hear her laugh.

Wanting to laugh for the same reason as she.

206 He had to put it together on his own. Walking along the road in front of the college one evening, he said, Wait a minute, you mean that…

And she said, Yes.

All three of them?

Yes.

207 The laugh delves deeper than history or circumstance. It comes from a world more real than, but inclusive of, the world of streets and houses where they walk.

To hear her tell, her family and home life is nothing out of the ordinary.

She has entered a reality where mother and father are left behind, where brothers and sister separate, where a child raises herself, where the body is broken from birth, where a child born to one is raised by another, where there is more than just the possibility of laughter, and the laughter is divine.

208 *You're not getting bashful now, are you, Johnny?*

Yes. No. I'll say it: *I believe in the resurrection of the body.* The words have a resonance now that they did not have when I heard and said them aloud with everyone else, each Sunday, from a very young age. You heard them too, over the speakerphone hookup to the church. What did you think? What *do* you think? I'm assuming there would be some modification to the body.

Johnny wants to give us a make-over.

Though I would not have wanted it any other way. I would not have wanted not to know you exactly as you were. I would not like to lose even a moment of your slow decline.

Don't lose your grip now, Johnny.

209 It comes up, but not often.

It came up unexpectedly in conversation. A friend put Mary Ann on the spot one evening, asking her to tell the others in the room about her family.

Later he explained that he felt he could do so because the longer we knew each other as friends the more interwoven our lives were becoming.

"Your brothers are part of my story now too," he said.

210 *Dear God, you're kidding.* This is the usual response, the historical response when people first hear that all three of Mary Ann's brothers died in their late teens or early twenties, within six months of each other, of the disease with which they were born.

It is a bit much to take in, in one sentence. And one reason why we tell the tale so infrequently.

Few people, in the subsequent overwhelming of their emotions, register the sentence that follows the first. Or maybe they just find it too hard to believe.

She and I have gone through the boxes in the basement together, paged through the photo albums, watched slides on the wall, discovered details of her family life either forgotten or never known. She didn't realize what good taste in clothing her mother had. She would especially like to have one of Fran's overcoats from the 1950s.

Mary Ann has read through these pages. She has added and subtracted. A private person, she is nonetheless willing to live with the feeling of being "outed."

What you have to understand, after the bald facts, the one-sentence summary, is that it was all *good.*

211 She is too well-acquainted with death.
What happened to her family, to her, never ceases to be unfair.

212 When Paul died, the story was about a disease that had taken the life of a young man.
    The story was of a brother who lost his best friend.
    When Eric died the story repeated, ramified.
    When Neil died, the story was about three brothers who died within half a year. The story was about parents who had lost all three of their sons.
    When Boss died, a wife and mother who had lost her three boys and had just begun to put her married life back together, lost her husband.
    When Mumphy died, the story became the daughter who lost her entire family: three brothers, father and mother.
    The stories do not cancel or replace each other. They are family.

213   UNCARVED TOTEMS

Coming here today, still thinking of Anastasia,
who died, too slowly, half-paralyzed, poor rat,
dragging herself across the cage. A pet's
old age: interminably brief.
                    Built a box,
white pine, at last: long having wanted
to build one they might break out of, if life
rebreathed – or wait: it would return with them
to earth: same gift.

Wrapped it
down in the roots of the Flowering Plum.

Come, let us share our dead.
Animal. Personal.

Walking here, by Aberdeen,
Longwood Road, those raw old barkless columns of pine
occur. This one, then, stands for Anastasia,
thanks, who with the others, if you eyeball
down the street, is faithfully propping up
its sagging piece of sky. That's so the roof
won't fall in, again, though if feels like it has,
at first – it always feels like it has. But
they keep it up, the dead. They lean
this way and that, twist in and out
of our line of vision, but they're still employed,
these poles, these uncarved totems,
who stand for them.

And them's many.
The war goes, but undeclared, not well.
Taking the shortcut here, the count
is already more than my recall: a few
aunts, uncles rarely met, the grandparents
on her side, and mine. Her father –
his heart attack, vacationing
in his homeland, overseas; and his sons,
her brothers, all three, who died too slowly
of their disease, which he by awful graciousness
had lived just long enough to see.
A person could learn to hate

these inborn muscular ironies, that push
and bully our simple intricate lives.
And she carries it yet, that part of her
that splintered when they broke away;
and one of the poles we go by
stands for her. The one, perhaps,
you saw me lean against, remembering this,
inventing, pretending
something to say.

                    They age in the elements,
these poles, these posts, these trunks of pine
stripped of all their clothing.
They line the way, stand by
to haul our messages, communicate
the latest or the last reports, to bear
our sometime recognition, grief and memory,
our invitation over the same earth we travel
coming to this place,
                    to give them name,
to share
            our deaths,
            who go,
                    who also stay.

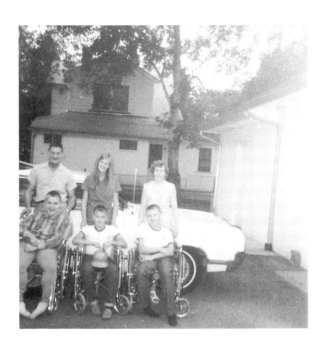

NOTES

Sections 4, 29, 37, 66, 73, 80, 183 and 188 are copyright © Mary Terpstra, 2005.

Sections 32, 35 & 47 are quotations from "Professional Guide to Diseases," 1982.

Section 75 mentions a list that Fran made of those who came to the house as friends and neighbours, practical nurses, homemakers, bringers of tapes, magazines and papers, evening help, feeders & exercise people. The names on that list were: Annajean Leegwater, Clareen Vanden Berg, Emma Jones, Mamie Allen, Janine Floyd, Diane Ryan, Phyllis Schipper, Rosemary Di Metrio, Helen Fazio, Carmella, Eleanor Schneidenbach, Catherine Tanan, Catherine Tchinnis, Mary Ishii, Henry Abma, David Schipper, Rick Tuit, Dennis Leegwater, Larry Brandes, Paul Brinkerhoff, John Bookis, Mark Plowman, Henry Van Wageningen, Neil Van Wageningen, John Van Wageningen, Johan Van Wageningen, John Brinkerhoff, Karen Holmes, Joyce Hammett, Lorraine Gruber, Diane Hoffman, Herm Hagedorn, Siebenn Spoelstra, Diane Hagedorn, Mieke Bandstra, Nancy Simcox, Ann Smith, Nancy Clement, Henriette Borst, Jane Malefyt, Gertrude Borst, Eleanor Snyder, Janet Hogg, Ellen Chase, Carol De Vries, Nell Kerlen, Norma McDonald, Eleanor Jeltes, Helen Godfrey, Betty Block, Alice Valkema, Martha De Hoog, Thea Leegwater, Jean Abma, Polly Baker, Jean Woudenberg, Kathy Voorman, Wilma Dykhouse, Janice Bandstra, Angie Van Dongen, Jane Brinkerhoff and Ruth Knyfd.

Section 162 is "Scrabbling for Repose," from *Scrabbling for Repose* by John Terpstra (Toronto: Split Reed Press, 1982).

Section 165 is quoted from a talk Barbara Brown Taylor delivered at Calvin College, Grand Rapids, MI, in April 2004.

Section 213 is "Uncarved Totems," from *The Church Not Made with Hands* by John Terpstra (Toronto: Wolsak & Wynn, 1997).

An excerpt from this book originally appeared in *Image*.

Gaspereau Press acknowledges the support of the Canada Council for the Arts, the Nova Scotia Department of Tourism & Culture, and the Government of Canada through the Book Publishing Industry Development Program.

Typeset in Quadraat and Quadraat Sans by Andrew Steeves and printed offset and bound at Gaspereau Press, Kentville, Nova Scotia. The figures reproduced on the cover are after paper cut-outs made by John Terpstra. The photograph is from the collection of John and Mary Terpstra.

9 8 7 6 5 4 3 2 1

Library and Archives Canada Cataloguing in Publication

Terpstra, John
The boys, or, Waiting for the electrician's daughter
/ John Terpstra.
ISBN 1-55447-011-0

1. Muscular dystrophy – Patients – Biography. I. Title.
II. Title: Waiting for the electrician's daughter.
RC935.M7T47 2005   362.196'748'00922   C2005-903605-2

GASPEREAU PRESS PRINTERS & PUBLISHERS
47 CHURCH AVENUE, KENTVILLE, NOVA SCOTIA
CANADA B4N 2M7   WWW.GASPEREAU.COM